Ask the Right Question

Luigi Bandini Buti

Ask the Right Question

A Rational Approach to Design for All in Italy

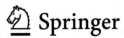 Springer

Luigi Bandini Buti
Faculty of Design
Polytechnic University of Milan
Milan, Italy

ISBN 978-3-030-07178-3   ISBN 978-3-319-96346-4   (eBook)
https://doi.org/10.1007/978-3-319-96346-4

This Springer imprint is published by the registered company Springer Nature Switzerland AG
The registered company address is: Gewerbestrasse 11, 6330 Cham, Switzerland

Foreword I

According to Eurostat, some 70 million European (circa 21% of the population) was aged 60 or more in 1997. As we live longer lives and the birth rate continues to fall, more than 35% of Europe's population will be aged 60 or more by 2020, net of immigration.

Years ago, I happened to be talking to a member of the D2 unit at the European Commission's Directorate-General for Enterprise, who was responsible for drawing up a discussion paper on user-driven innovation.

We discussed how we could learn about future consumers' needs and aspirations, including the ones they may perceive but about which they are not yet fully aware. We concluded that the answer was to put together groups of consumers and ask them the right questions.

And now I have in my hands the proofs of a book written by Luigi Bandini Buti about this very concept of asking the right question: an exhaustive manual, written in that inimitable style of yours that disseminates with a smile, yet is no less rigorous for that. Drawing on the principles of Design for All, it makes another contribution to spreading knowledge about the many and varied applications of this meritorious tool for social integration.

Thank you, Gino.

Rodrigo Rodriquez
www.rodrigorodriquez.com

Foreword II

In times of great technological transformations and digital ubiquity, many of us find ourselves wondering how much longer it will be before we interact with robots or cyborgs at every moment in our everyday lives, the kind of thing we see in the movies.

Today's increasing levels of automation will oblige us to refashion the meaning of our existence, both personal and with regard to our work, so as to be able to live in a world with increasingly innovative, customised products and services designed so that any individual can use them with comfort.

In other words, although technology has great opportunities to give us, it is always the human being who should direct the necessary developments and dominate the environment that surrounds him, by making a careful analysis of his needs.

Although at first sight it may not appear to be directly pertinent to the technological context of our age, the repeated reference to a humanistic approach that comes across in this book by Luigi Bandini Buti actually furnishes us with the magnifying glass wielded by the alert observer, the expert who studies civil society and can help us understand how human existence has to interface increasingly with changes that are not restricted to technology alone, but also encompass the individual and the social context in which he expresses himself and relates to others.

"Ask the Right Question" captures the essence of how to interpret the events of our times correctly and provides us with the right approach for disseminating wellness in such a way that it will be increasingly equitably distributed among human beings: the level of technology that we have achieved will enable us to live longer and better-quality lives, adapt our homes as well as our factories and offices and interconnect with the objects we own, all with increasing ease.

I believe that the path mapped out here by Luigi Bandini Buti is the right one, also for adapting technology to suit the needs of micro-firms and craft businesses. The implementation of a humanistic approach with the potential to generate an increasing flow of advantages for the individual, in fact, also paves the way for a greater convergence between such firms and large-scale industry in terms of technology.

On the other hand, contexts of innovation are destined to open up increasingly as a consequence of the input of experts specialised in a variety of disciplines. And Design for All will enable micro-firms operating in many fields (construction, wood and furnishings, complements, accessories, etc.) to express their voices more effectively in polyvalent functional groups partnering with external experts from the professions, the universities and technological backgrounds.

In short, if the collaborative approach is combined with the humanistic approach to design, it can enable the specific skills necessary for creating a new product or service to be recognised, facilitated and strengthened, also in terms of a network approach to firms, which can have a far greater impact than the one that used to treat innovation as something that happened within the confines of individual businesses.

It is a question of establishing a method of design and of corporate development inspired by a logic that in some respects makes a clean break with the past, but this path is one that we shall have to tread if Italy's micro-firms, so inextricably related to our country's history, are to be able to take advantage of many promising market niches in the near future.

Co-working, fablabs and social agriculture are just three examples of how social and participatory innovation are evolving into one of the driving forces of new economic initiatives. This is not a question of promoting top-down forms of inclusion, but of developing bottom-up initiatives that create a level playing field for everyone. Design for All enables this to be achieved, since it throws light on how to go about designing, from the very start, products and services for a broad spectrum of individuals, using what technology has to offer to cater for people's real needs.

Rovigo, Italy   Andrea Scalia
                                                          Innovation and Networking,
                                                            Confartigianato Firms

Preface

This book is the result of experience of working with Confartigianato in Vicenza, whose aim was to train technicians at all levels to be capable of catering for the needs of the elderly. To achieve this, a course was organised that attracted the participation of many firms, designers, plant installers and social and health professionals, who for various reasons all took an interest in accessible housing. Avril Accolla and I, as lecturers, realised that it was far from easy to convey the notions in question appropriately to people with such widely different backgrounds, curricula and interests, so we devised a multicultural system that we decided to call "Ask the Right Question".[1]

Milan, Italy   Luigi Bandini Buti

---

[1] Translator's note: What the Italian title recommends is in fact that you, the designer, should actually "ask *yourself* the right question" (my italics). In Italian, the phrase trips off the tongue very easily, more easily, indeed, than the phrase "ask the right question", but it is altogether more of a mouthful in English. Since the author has used the title repeatedly throughout his book, quoting it as the name that he gives to a model of investigation, I chose to leave the reflexive part of the verb out of the title, on the understanding with the author that I would explain this choice at the earliest opportunity.

Translator's Note

Every translator who sets out to tackle a new text has to make a fundamental decision about the approach to be adopted in his work, because there are more ways than one of going about the task.

The accuracy and consistency of technical language and terminology are unquestionably of paramount importance in scientific and academic texts, since scholars from different linguistic and cultural backgrounds will descend on the new contribution and pick it to pieces, take exception to it, quote it and derive further reasoning from the positions it adopts and the motives it cites for adopting them. In such cases, it is understandable that accuracy of linguistic rendering from one medium to another is of such all-pervading significance as to relegate such issues as readability and the ability to hold the reader's interest to a secondary level, if indeed they are even taken into consideration at all. Such is the price society sometimes pays for the continuous flow of academic discussion.

Yet for all its decades of practical impact in the real world, design is still a relative newcomer to the world of academia: while it has certainly laboured to establish a viable lexicon of its own that lexicon, together with the grammar used in its expression, has to reflect the idiosyncratic development of the discipline, which does not owe the development of its writings to the solitary strivings of academics slaving away in the rarefied atmospheres of hermetically-sealed faculties, but to the jottings and reflections of professionals who spend most of their days working as creatives in the market, ever in search of innovative solutions for tackling the issues that a rapidly-changing society turns up in sometimes quite unexpected places and at quite unexpected times.

Design theory and its writings are one of those hybrid creatures that are born when real-world experience (in this case, of design practice) comes face-to-face with the need to record it in a manner that academia may (at times begrudgingly) acknowledge. Clearly, these writings are unlikely to be couched in a strictly academic language, and it is the responsibility of the translator to take due note and act accordingly.

In addition to all this, it has been my great privilege to count the author of this book, Luigi Bandini Buti (Gino his friends), among my close personal friends for some fifteen years. Fifteen years in which we have worked together closely in furthering the cause of the theory and practice of Design for All, both in Italy, where we both live, and internationally: fifteen years of intense and always fruitful discussions, that enable me to say, not without a note of pride, that I understand how his mind works.

Gino is a native of the northern Italian region of Emilia Romagna, where storytelling has long developed as a fine art. Like many a creative, but in practice better than most, Gino is himself a past master at storytelling, highly skilled at framing complex issues in parables that render their complexity instantly comprehensible, also for the layman with no particularly highly developed background in the lexicon of design theory.

My aim in translating this book into English has been twofold: (1) to ensure that the meaning, and not just the strict wording, of the message conveyed by Gino is communicated faithfully to his readers in another idiom, while at the same time ensuring academic substance and consistency of terminology and (2) to capture and reproduce, in a different language, the always serious—yet sometimes also playful —tone of the original and above all of its author. My hope is that the result does not read like an academic tome, but like the tales of a lifetime of experience being told by a friendly older mentor, for that is what it should be.

Pete Kercher

Acknowledgements

This book was written as a result of a close working relationship with Avril Accolla.

For their help in writing the definitive version of the book, my thanks go to Pete Kercher for his perspicacious translation, to Gregorio Strano for his assistance, to my children Cristina and Simone for their relations and to everyone else who gave me advice.

Contents

Part I
Background

Chapter 1
Design for All

Products, places and systems should be developed to cater for all individuals.

A little while ago, a young colleague asked me: "Since you take an interest in these things, can you tell me what kitchen is best suited to a person who has to use a wheelchair?" He had been commissioned to adapt a flat to the new requirements of a client who had come out of hospital, but in a wheelchair.

I gave him some information about what the market had to offer for people with disabilities.

He was back on the telephone a few days later, apologising for having to disturb me again, but this time he wanted to know my opinion: what would it be better to use in that project, gas burners or an induction hob? I was happy to answer him with all my professional experience: gas burners make it really evident to the user when they are on or off and also how intensely they are being used, but they are not easy to clean. They are also intrinsically dangerous because they rely on using gas, even though today's protection systems are very effective. An induction hob is very easy to clean, but the message it sends about whether it is on or off is not natural (like the gas flame), but codified (you have to read signs and symbols). And it is not suitable for all pans. You cannot use a wok, with its rounded base, for example. "Is your client a good cook, someone who cares about his kitchen?" I asked.

I immediately realised that my question had embarrassed him: "Actually... I don't know", he answered.

"What do you mean 'you don't know'? Who are you designing this kitchen for?"

"I know he is in a wheelchair, so I have to make him a kitchen for a disabled user."

He had already told me that his client lived with his family, so there was no guarantee that he himself would be doing the cooking. "You know, before you make any decisions, you have to ask yourself some questions", I advised him, then went on to tell him that he needed to know how his client related to the kitchen before the event that had disabled him: was he a skilled chef, someone who often cooked himself, or was there someone else in the family who prepared the food? And if he was not the one who did the cooking, did he have to prepare his own food under certain circumstances, such as during his or his relatives' holidays? Or did he need no more than a coffee and a fried egg? If we were in the USA, his culinary

© Springer Nature Switzerland AG 2019
L. Bandini Buti, *Ask the Right Question*,
https://doi.org/10.1007/978-3-319-96346-4_1

needs would most probably go little further than owning a can opener and a microwave! But that would never be enough here in Italy... luckily!

Once you know about the past, I continued, the next thing is to find out what has changed. Maybe nothing will alter about the way he lived his life beforehand, or will there be changes?

You have to ask questions; but what's more, you have to ask the right questions.

Only after you have asked those questions can you start thinking about the solutions, which might be the creation of a kitchen suitable for a person in wheelchair, following the principle that he has few or no opportunities to adapt, while the other members of his family have far more. But it might also be a 'normal' kitchen where it is also possible for a wheelchair user to make himself a coffee without any difficulty; or it might be a kitchen that pays no particular attention to the wheelchair user, because he will never be able to use it or even want to, because he cannot or because he is assisted at all times.

By now it should be clear to everyone that the statement "...he is in a wheelchair, so I have to make him a kitchen for a disabled user" risks being dangerous nonsense.

A good design, a design for everyone, relies on us asking the right questions before we make any decisions. That is what we are taught by Design for All, which also stipulates that the questions are not just a pleasant opportunity to have some contact with reality, but must be structured to be effective, efficient and satisfactory.

***

Mankind's artefacts have to provide responses to the needs, aspirations and dreams of those who use them.

But how do we go about getting to know what they are?

We have to ask the people who know!

Good design theory and practice teach us that anyone who sets out to develop a design certainly asks questions and looks for answers: questions and answers concerned with people, what they need, the tools they have and how they use them, what they know and what they dream about, the context, the environment and the market.

Products, places and systems also have to cater for people with sensory, perceptive and cognitive limitations. Not just the ones that are obvious, whether permanent or temporary, but also the ones we have because of a moment of distraction, inexperience, tiredness or anything else.

It is no easy challenge.

It takes more than a good designer's common sense or the use of common knowledge to tackle this task appropriately. The designer will need to get access to specific and often specialised information, such as in the area of physical and biological impairments. A superficial smattering of various disciplines will almost never be sufficient: you will need to learn the skill of involving other disciplines and other people, some of them with a high degree of specialisation.

That is why there is a need for this specialised toolkit to help you "ask the right questions".

THINKING ABOUT IT

When I studied, immediately after the Second World War, there were none of the disciplines that we cannot and must not do without these days. For example, the first talk about sociology and psychology was quite timid, partly because they had been ostracised in Italy by fascism, which knew what role people were supposed to have: men were supposed to become good soldiers (and obey the state) and women were supposed to do the housework and have lots of children (and obey their husbands). In the case of objects, it was already a miracle if they functioned, if they moved: who cared about safety or comfort?

So when I studied, I found myself having to take care of everything myself: I had to be a technician, a psychologist, a sociologist, a doctor and more besides. And all of it was rather superficial, of course.

These days, our society expects specialised input and it is not enough to read things up in books and magazines. Today's culture is one of complexity. Today's cars are no simple self-propelling vehicles any more (in the old days, they just had to move!), but objects that are fully integrated into everyone's lives, offering high performance, comfort and safety, which all means a great deal to people's sense of status.

1.1 In Praise of Diversity

Diversity is a resource.

The title "In Praise of Diversity" is a little pretentious. I trust that Erasmus would excuse me, but the Design for All philosophy does indeed state that diversity is a resource. We do not need to disturb Darwin to know that diversity is the driver of evolution and of change. I first said this myself in 2010.[1]

THINKING ABOUT IT

I asked a musician friend of mine how come symphony orchestras always have so many musicians, with all the costs and organisation that involves. I asked him why, for example, the twenty violins in an orchestra cannot be replaced by taking just one violin and amplifying it twenty times or by reproducing the sound of one violin through twenty loudspeakers. He explained that the quality of the orchestra's sound comes from its diversity, from the imperceptible differences between one instrument and another and between one violinist and another. *It's the diversity that makes the orchestra.*

I think it is fair to say that our age has discovered diversity, after wasting so much time pointlessly trying to treat everybody as though we were all the same. Just look at what happened to those regimes that set out to abolish difference, by forcing people to adopt the same habits, models, behaviour and identical uniforms for everyone. The only one left is North Korea. They did not treat diversity as a resource, but as a problem. But their people are diverse and want to be.

---

[1]L. Bandini Buti in "Elogio della diversità - La pratica del Design for All trasforma la diversità in una risorsa" (In Praise of Diversity: How the practice of Design for All transforms diversity into a resource), round table organised by Design for All Italia in the Palazzo dei Mercanti, Milan, 9 October 2010, in the framework of the Innovation Festival.

Of course, diversity can also be inconvenient. What does it mean to design for individuals who are all diverse? Remember what Henry Ford said? "You can have your car in any colour you want, so long as it's black".

1.2   Design for All

If it is true that diversity is a resource and a characteristic of our times, then design has to take that into account.

These days all the human disciplines recognise that diversity is intrinsic to human beings and that we are lucky that this is so. Yet diversity seems to clash with the demand for mass production to be standardised. It would be so much easier to design just one product that would be good for everyone: the users would then have to adapt! But that is actually rather silly and stupid: the real world is not like that.

The new frontier of design is to treat diversity as a resource, because it is from such challenges that innovation comes. Yet achieving design for diversity is far from being a walkover, since it seems to contradict production's need for serial systems. But if we manage to design "for All", we can expand the market base.

THINKING ABOUT IT

Here is an example. Some Swedish students of mine were telling me about the cheese slice that is apparently an indispensable piece of kitchenware in their country, just like the cheese grater is for us in Italy, where we grate Parmesan. The cheese slice has always had a horizontal handle like a potato peeler, obliging the user to adopt an unnatural posture of the wrist. Research aimed at catering for a niche of people who have a hand-grip disability suggested designing a cheese slice with a vertical handle. This soon became people's favourite configuration as the object became popular and was copied, because it was simply more comfortable for everyone. It took a higher-than-usual level of attention and an interdisciplinary approach to get a somnolent market to move. In this case, the disability proved itself to be a commercial resource.

Industrial production prefers serial systems and standardisation, while product differentiation is intrinsic to craftsmanship and the quest for repetition always looks rather forced.

The question now is what the spread of the new 3D printing technology will bring.

At least in theory, the economies of scale and replication will be flanked by a market of small numbers and diversity. The future may hold products that are turned out in small or even tiny series, or even adapted by the end user to suit his specific needs. The place where the production takes place may be remote, as what moves will be the design, in the form of software.

THINKING ABOUT IT

One excellent example of what 3D printing technologies mean today can be found in the "e-NABLING the future" project, a community that manages the possibility to amend and print artificial hands for children on an open-source basis. High-performance artificial hands are already available on the market, but children grow quickly and need a new one every six months. You can imagine what that costs. But with 3D printing, the changeover is made much easier and cheaper. Everybody uses a network of data and contributes, so that the network is enriched each time by their own experience. We shall be seeing a lot more developments in this field.

The process of designing any tangible or intangible artefact should always take place in reference to what the people who will use it actually need—and that includes their need for things to be pleasant and for their dreams to be respected. To achieve this, we have to know the needs, aspirations and dreams of all those people who can reasonably be expected to come into contact with the product. This is a quite delicate activity that calls for us to think and act in a structured manner if we are to achieve it.

This is the aim of the "Ask the right question" methodology.

THINKING ABOUT IT

If we look at the mediaeval cathedrals, we notice that the architectural elements are all different from one another. The building's general structure was co-ordinated by a master mason applying the knowledge acquired by the community, then the details (such as the capitals) were entrusted to specialised masons who were given specific theological topics to express: here we shall illustrate the work done in the seasons, there the theological virtues and so on. I recently had the opportunity to study the façade of the collegiate church of Casauria, near Pescara, where I observed basket capitals, like in Ravenna, capitals inspired by the Corinthian style and innovative capitals that had certainly been designed by Teutonic masons, all one next to the other. What a creative ferment! (And what a denial of the idea of the "Dark Ages"). It shows the power of imagination and diversity. But then along came Brunelleschi (the first architect in the modern sense of the term), who imposed the details for the church of Santo Spirito in Florence, insisting that all the altars should be identical to his designs, so the masons went on strike. It was the beginning of the division in the modern era between those who design and those who execute the designs.

1.3 Decision-Makers

Designers must have the capacity to design for the future.

The designer has a set of objectives for which the product he is designing must cater, objectives that he has set for himself or that have been provided by a client. He has been told that his design must cater for certain specific requirements, which are conveyed to him in accordance with the logic and the language of marketing or of technological opportunities. The designer has to interpret them using the language of design.

THINKING ABOUT IT

What should a product dedicated to young women be like, for example? Do designers know how to make their designs cater for this issue?

We can do better than simply saying that it does not necessarily have to be pink, because pink is the supposedly typical feminine colour. But there is a real risk of a tendency to think that if you know all there is to know about the market, then you already have all the knowledge about this issue that you need: all you have to do is look at what has already been done and make it better! In other words: look at the past to design for the future. Which is evidently a contradiction. The issue is what will appeal to young women and, even if the designer is a young woman herself, while she will certainly know all about her own requirements and preferences, they are hers and hers alone. So she does not in fact know about what other young women require and prefer: while there will certainly be some common ground, they will have their own individual needs, aspirations and dreams. But there's more: what problems will those young women have to face tomorrow, when the product is on the market? Will Barbie have become a thing of the past?

Projections and intuitions simply are not enough.

The best source of information is the person for whom the designer is designing the product. And the best way to unearth this information is through market surveys that tell us a great deal about that person's habits and behaviour under certain circumstances, as well as how such events are distributed statistically.

But they tell us very little about more subjective things. For example, should the product you are about to create come across in terms of its efficiency, its playfulness or its wow factor? But above all: how should it encapsulate these sensations?

Let's take a rather obvious example. If you want to create an inclusive individual means of personal movement (another way of saying a wheelchair), it really should not look as if it just came out of a hospital. But what is it that gives a product that hospital, domestic or sports flavour? Creatives are expected to answer this question, although they will have a hard time finding anything in the market surveys.

Getting to know these issues of fundamental importance for developing a design is never an easy business. If you ask potential users directly, you may not get reliable answers, as they might not be able to answer you in terms of the kind of information you need and, when they do answer you, you would not know how to weight each individual's answers. To what model does the individual refer when expressing abstract concepts? You don't know what conceptual benchmarks he uses: does the word 'luxury' mean expensive, exclusive or the kind of thing that is used every day by VIPs? Every one of us has his own yardstick and it is difficult to identify and compare them.

THINKING ABOUT IT

Many researchers tend to ask interviewees about what products should be like if they are to cater for their needs. That is the worst approach to adopt!

Individuals are only capable of providing reliable responses based on their own current experience: they are not capable of imagining future models. Here is an example: what answers would we have received in 1990 if we had asked people what they thought of a strictly two-seater car available for the price of a four-seater? The answers would certainly have been a thinly-veiled rebuff. But that car is now on the streets: the Smart constitutes a new concept of mobility!

And what about the difficulties encountered in introducing full electric vehicles, which are still seen today as a niche for rich enthusiasts. Since that translates into hesitation that the market will not accept them, they tend to be launched as luxury saloon cars, complete with a large volume at the front where the engine used to be... although it is now completely empty. In design terms, it's nothing short of insulting.

Another issue that is dear to Design for All is that of involving the entire value chain. Are good designers a must if you want your trains to be better suited to today's requirements? Of course they are: but if those who manage the transport system do not decide that now is the time to change, nothing at all will happen. So the first people you have to approach with these issues are the decision-makers at the top of the tree, regardless of whether they are in the public or the private sector.

Every design starts with a brief, i.e. with a declaration of the objectives, a description of the issue to be tackled, any limitations, the time frame and the means available. Irrespective of whether the proposal comes from a client or is at the designer's own initiative, it is the result of quite precise research, planning, intuition and/or input that cannot and must not be questioned.

Indeed, the designer must abide by the brief scrupulously, but can and must also enrich it.

A good designer must never be a passive actor, but should always propose an 'expanded brief', i.e. go in search of design features that can be adopted without contradicting or disfiguring the premises of the original brief, so as to achieve a significant expansion of the product's use (alterations and/or additions that call for a small investment and have a minor technical impact, but a major effect in terms of expansion of the product's usage). A good designer may also look on the brief as the 'generator of a family', i.e. consider how the design, once developed, may become the starting point for other products for uses that were not originally envisaged, exploiting the economies of scale, for example as a way of making niche products more competitive.

THINKING ABOUT IT

When designing a table for communities, it is possible to make provision—at little or no extra cost—for legs that double as hooks for bags and handbags, with protected or protectable edges to ensure child safety and other such features. The folding back seat of a family car can be divided in two in such a way as to make space for skis or a surfboard, creating a city car where the surfboard also has its place, because, after all, some cities are located by the sea. These are all low-cost ideas that relate to uses not expressed in the brief.

Electric golf caddies and the vehicles used by the post office or the police lend themselves to being generators of families of vehicles for exploring tourist venues, historical gardens and so on.

A design should not cater for the past, nor even the present, but must look to the future. A certain amount of time passes between the moment of any product's conception and when it is launched on to the market. In the case of architectural products, years may pass between the definition of the city plan and moment when the buildings it envisaged are actually used for the first time. In the case of a car, the time lapse between conception and production is generally from three to five years, after which it has to stay up-to-date for many more years.

Chapter 2
Ask the Right Question
(A Design System)

Formulating the right question is already part of the design process.

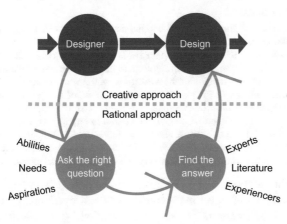

"Ask the right question" is an approach to the design process that draws a distinction between the moment when information is gathered (which takes the shape of formulating the right questions and seeking answers) and the actual creative design process.

Gathering information is a rational approach that draws on all the disciplines and techniques available for assessing and measuring phenomena. The design process is a creative approach that draws on humanistic disciplines.

So is there really a need for a new model of approach?

I think there is. "Ask the right question" says that the first creative act of a design process lies deciding in how to formulate the questions. The answers are drawn from the huge sea of information, questioning people directly, consulting the literature or involving experts. What you get is a mass of knowledge, all of it true, but often inconsistent or contradictory, that calls for a critical organisation of the thinking that will lead the designer to make the creative decisions that are his specific input. Those decisions can often be quite painful, as they rule out everything that is discarded, as well as exciting, because they contain creation.

© Springer Nature Switzerland AG 2019
L. Bandini Buti, *Ask the Right Question*,
https://doi.org/10.1007/978-3-319-96346-4_2

2.1   The Phases of Design for All

No information is automatically design. No computer can replace creativity.

"Ask the right question" sets out to organise how information is gathered, so that the designer does not have to rely on his own sensitivity, but can also draw on a guide to organise his thinking.

The first act in a design process is finding out. If you want to find out, you have to ask yourself questions. The right questions lead to answers. But it is not easy to ask the right questions: it means having ideas about how needs develop, having identified the intersections of individuals' lives and how they think, their past and their probable future, and also having identified technical developments and their trends.

THINKING ABOUT IT

When you work with firms that operate in the market, there is often no provision made for the time (and the means) for gathering information. The time available is often dictated by external deadlines, special occasions in the market or something else. This means that there is a temptation to feel obliged to skip any form of investigation and base everything on your own intuition (to the eternal joy of the academics, who favour getting things right formally over actual feasibility). But if you are thinking in terms of Design for All, the aim is to improve the quality of life for everyone, also at the price of formal simplification. Many authors have stated that the first people interviewed in any investigation will already give you up to 90% of the right answers and the number you have to interview to build on that percentage increase exponentially. So even only 5–10 interviewees will already give you a strong orientation... sowing confusion even among the pure academics.

Every right question must be addressed to the right person and in the right way.

The answers, which are often contradictory and overlapping, have to be taken together to get the framework of knowledge that will guide the designer in making his creative design decisions.

If you fail to apply a certain, transmittable philosophical design structure, you run the risk of getting solutions that are partly ineffective, insufficient or improvised.

THINKING ABOUT IT

Some time ago, I wrote a short essay called *Heavy is Beautiful*. These days, light is beautiful.

When I was a boy, I had the adventure of working as mechanic for a summer in my uncle's workshop in Romagna. That's where I learned what a car was in those days. My uncle would take a carburettor and adapt it to another type of car to make it more powerful or transform it, and he did the same with the distributor or the silencer. At the end of the war, we were lucky if we had plenty of leftover parts that we could put together to invent some rickety machinery for sawing wood or flushing out cesspits. But how many people know how a motor is made these days? It's become a mysterious object: perfect, but mysterious. In those days, you could tell a complex mechanism from its basic components and the object's final form reflected how they were assembled together. The spare wheel was mounted outside the car and the headlights were screwed onto the mudguards.

What radically changed our ability to understand how things function was the advent of information technology. Before then, a heavy object was worth more than a light one: it contained more material and that meant more substance and more work, so would be more effective. But that's not how things are today. It will not be long before we even have a computer under our skin. We already have pacemakers there!

The days are over when a good designer could have a complete overview of technical, human and market issues. These days, complexity and specialisation are inalienable factors that call for far more input than the designer's intuition alone.

THINKING ABOUT IT

"Ask the right question" can become a mass academic and scientific product that, since it is an intrinsically simple tool, enables everyone involved in the design process to use it: not just designers, but decision-makers, managers, maintenance staff etc. And that, too, is what makes it modern.

2.2   Asking the Right Question Is the First Important Act in the Design Process

"To design things, you have to start out from people, not things."

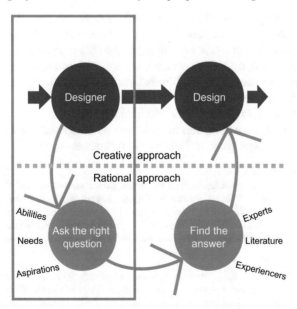

Before they get down to work on any kind of design process, designers have to gather information.

They have to know the purpose of the project, what place it will occupy in the market, its outlines and what has already been done in the field, so as to avoid repeating it or to make use of its experience, plus how free they are to operate and any restrictions, relevant technologies, costs and more besides.

Nobody would dream of doubting that they have to ask questions.

What's not so obvious is what tools are available for formulating the questions. Of course it's important to draw on your own professionality and the experience that enables you to find your way around what you have already done, but that may be misleading if you want to innovate. Analysing what others have done before you may also lead you to believe that it is correct (...that's the way that people have always done it!), but it may be a trap, because it gives you the impression that you are right... but in fact you are only living in the past.

Design theories offer us subjective investigations that are actually a great tool for gathering knowledge, but only if you are capable of distinguishing between there here and now (which it is possible to investigate thoroughly) and the future, which is never a mere extrapolation and calls for a conceptual elaboration that is often anything but straightforward.

THINKING ABOUT IT

Designers often furnish their own answers. They may be tempted to think that if something works for them as human beings, then it will work for everyone.

Nothing could be further from the truth!

Every one of us is unique, with our pros and cons, our interests, knowledge, habits etc. And they are certainly not the same as everyone else's. Luckily: otherwise we would all be robots.

A designer may tend to discard the questions whose answers do not occur to him in advance, along with the ones that seem to be absurd or contradictory.

If we analyse a tool like a mobile telephone, it's immediately obvious that the keys have to be big enough to ensure that large or trembling fingers do not press two of them at the same time, but it's also obvious that the telephone has to be small enough to fit in a pocket.

So we need big keys on a small mobile telephone!

It seems to be a contradiction in terms and designers may be tempted to ignore the problem and paper it over. But both requirements are true.

THINKING ABOUT IT

There came a time when the mobile telephone manufacturers realised the difficulty of having to produce, store and distribute different keyboards for different alphabets and languages (if you ever studied French at school, do you remember all those infuriating accents?): they had to sacrifice the size of the display to provide space for the keyboard (just as the boom of images was arriving) and still had tight, undersized keyboards.

Then along came the touchscreen and it was a revolution.

The manufacturers could now produce virtual keyboards with variable dimensions and contents that appear and disappear as you need them. The cost of storage has been reduced drastically, because manufacturers no longer need to have telephones with French, Spanish, Russian, Chinese and other keyboards, since all that information is now contained in the software. And the keys can be big or small to suit the user's needs.

Yet at the same time manufacturers had to deal with the needs of blind users, who were excluded completely when the tactile keys were abolished! They tackled the challenge by introducing voice commands that are also useful for anyone who is driving: when you have to keep your eyes on the road at all times, it is as though you are blind to everything else.

A design should be considered to be the result of the commitment of the entire chain of decision-making and not only of the professionals who work with design (engineers, architects and designers).

"Ask the right question" sets out to orient the questions to be asked in such a way that they are consistent with the resources and the time available and with the aims of the project. Note that this means orienting the questions, not looking for the answers. All too often, designers look for the answers without having formulated the questions, because they take the questions for granted.

The "right question" must enable us to get a clear picture of who will be using the result of the design in future.

It may seem obvious, but in practice it is not.

The users who come to mind immediately are the ones to whom the producer intends to offer his product, object, place or system and that he therefore tries to pamper and seduce. They will certainly be its first targets, the people who go out and buy it and who use it frequently: in other words, the ones it was devised for.

THINKING ABOUT IT

For whom should taxis be designed? For the passenger who pays for the ride or the driver who bought the car and who lives and works in it, sometimes in the freezing cold or torrid heat? Or should it be designed to adorn the city?

Well for all of these, obviously!

But these types of people have different needs. If you hail a taxi in the street, you expect to find a product that is friendly and prepared to cater for your diversified material requirements (no barriers, comfortable seating, easy to get in and out, quiet enough to hold a conversation and so on). To adorn the city, it should convey a sense of being modern and visible, but not intrusive, while for the driver it should be able to protect him (from the cold, from the heat and from prowlers), while providing comfort and distraction while waiting etc. And these are just a few hurried impressions that help us understand that there is no single truth, but many different truths that have to be the object of the "right questions". And the first of those questions is to find out "who?".

But the principles of accessibility and of Design for All tell us that we also have to think about other users, the ones who are not pampered by the manufacturers, maybe because they do not constitute enormous market segments or because they are not the ones who make the decisions about what to buy. These are occasional users or people who may encounter some difficulty in using the object, as well as the people who produce it, handle it, maintain it and decommission it. The designer needs to ask questions to discover the needs, the abilities and also the dreams of all these people.

THINKING ABOUT IT

Twice every year, I have to adjust all the clocks in my home when we pass from standard time to daylight saving and back again. Every time, I have to dig out the instruction manuals, because each system has its own logic that would be simple enough if we were to use it often, but becomes mysterious if we only use it twice a year. Am I the one who is a bit slow, or is it the designer who has not bothered to think about the people who will be using his system, how, when and with what degrees of cognition? Repeating actions often helps us remember them, while sporadic use makes them mysterious. That is why the maintenance engineer or the specialist brings different cognitive tools to bear on a problem from those used by ordinary people to tackle the same issue. And this is something that we only discover if we identify the different kinds of people who are destined to interact with the product and define their certain or probable characteristics.

2.3   Who, What, How?

A Design for All must start out from the questions Who? What? How?

The issues that guide how we formulate the "right question" are concerned with the people to whom the design is targeted (the "who"), the issues to be tackled by the design (the "what") and the method for doing so (the "how").

THINKING ABOUT IT

I always repeat that to design means to innovate. In other words, it means thinking about what people will need in the future, because what we design today must have a life tomorrow and not only today.

I tell my students that, if they set themselves the aim of designing a chair and they only look at chairs that are excellent, maybe one by Gio Ponti, by one of the Castiglioni brothers or also one by Philippe Starck, then they will make a chair that will be a Gio Ponti, a Castiglioni or a Philippe Starck ... but it will only be a second-hand version. They may actually sell really well, because the way has been paved by the prototypes, but you can say goodbye to innovation. But if they ask themselves what it means to hold the body active yet at rest, if they ask about changing models of behaviour and changing approaches to aesthetics, in the end they will certainly make a chair... but one that's different, more up to date and for everyone.

Who?
Designing for All does not restrict your creativity. On the contrary: it stimulates it with new challenges.
The "who" are the people who come into contact with the product or place during its life cycle. They are the people who produce it, distribute it, buy it, use it, manage it and recycle or decommission it.

Take toys for small children, for example, which are bought by adults to be used by children, while a product for slightly older children may be bought by the children themselves, though probably not in the sense that the children will hand over the money themselves (children are past masters at manipulating their elders!).

So the first question we have to ask ourselves is who will use the product and how can we classify them.

THINKING ABOUT IT

You have to think about the people who will use your product as individuals, not as stereotypes: that means that they are people, not car drivers, pedestrians, people with disabilities and so on. In the real world, every individual has multiple personalities, depending on the angle from which you observe him: the same person may be a car driver, a husband, a father, a taxpayer, a patient and so on.

But to find your way through this, it is reasonable to look at these personalities one by one, grouping individuals together in simple conceptual categories in relation to how they interact with the world and to their abilities and limits.

The "who" might be:

- *an individual*

These are specific people who can be identified as individuals with a name and surname.

If I have to work on an apartment for a client who has asked me to draw up a design, I shall find myself face to face with a real person, with an identity of his own and clear individual conditions of life, health and social intercourse.

I may/must ask him questions about his aspirations, his habits and his resources. I may get to know his family and they may even invite me to dinner. I may/must make a home tailored to his needs, his resources and his dreams.

In such cases as this, we can get to know every detail of the individual's characteristics, propensities and shortcomings and also how they are likely to evolve.

- *specialised categories*

These are people who have certain characteristics with strong connotations.

If you are asked to design a home for people who suffer from Alzheimer's disease, for example, or a boxing gym or a set of surgical instruments, you cannot expect to get to know all the people on the receiving end of your work individually, but you can be sure that they will share certain well-defined and identifiable characteristics. These categories have strong connotations not only in terms of their physical aspects or abilities, but also and above all in terms of their awareness of belonging to a category. There is no doubt that a golfer, for example, has a quite particular conception of the world and approach to it, although he then jettisons it when he goes back home.

In such cases, individuals may have standardising characteristics with strong connotations (e.g. rugby players, street cleaners, paraplegics and so on) and cannot in fact *not* have them.

THINKING ABOUT IT

In the course of my long career, I once had the adventurous opportunity of dealing with what I call a 'superniche': the prefabricated structures used by the police and armed forces to practice sharpshooting. The category was so well refined that there was no room in the design for any doubts.

Even so, the manufacturers of these structures were thrown completely off balance when this purely masculine environment started being used by women, by female soldiers. What hygienic problems do women have? How do they relate to others? How do they behave? And what will the regulation military bra look like? This was one specialised category whose certainties were utterly demolished by modernity!

- *defined categories*

These are individuals who at certain moments and in certain situations share certain aspects that can be attributed to a category.

These tend to be everybody, but with at least one shared characteristic: people who use an ATM (because they have a bank account), people who drive cars (because they have a driving licence), people who use the internet (because they have a computer), school children (because they have clearly-identifiable classes based on their age), members of the armed forces (because they are adult, healthy and have clearly-defined tasks) etc.

In some and maybe many cases, it will only be possible to refer to stereotypes. A flat that was built to be rented out is likely to be based on the stereotype of an average family, with some children still living at home, even though this phenomenon is said to be risking extinction. Cars will try to comply as far as possible with the characteristics and needs of the users for whom they were made, in accordance with well-established stereotypes (working women, commuters, travelling salesmen etc.). In such cases, you cannot get to know the individuals, but you can get to know some of the characteristics that are common to the category and then base your decisions of these.

- *everyone*

These people are unidentifiable because the activity that concerns them is generic.

Who takes a tram? Everyone. Who goes to the park? Everyone. Who sits down? Everyone.

"'Everyone' covers the individuals who want to make independent use of the system and have the reasonable probability of doing so."[1]

Since everyone eats, eating is a general characteristic. But there are "people who eat spaghetti". Here in Italy's that's "everyone", but in other countries they would be specialised. Here in Italy, you are specialised if you are capable of using chopsticks, but in China that's normal. The reason why I am pointing this out is not to cause confusion among all those who are fond of rigid certainty, but to convey the idea how relative concepts can be and how useful it is to "ask the right question", so as to avoid falling into simple traps.

In cases such as these, we cannot set any limits, because we are talking about people who have characteristics typical of the human race, albeit with variables to those characteristics and individual or social limitations.

THINKING ABOUT IT

When I am lecturing, I have noticed that students nearly always on the one hand feel the need to design something very clearly defined, but on the other seem to feel unbearably restricted by having to think about the characteristics and needs of the people who will use their products.

---

[1]A. Accolla, *Design for All, Il progetto per individuo reale*, Franco Angeli, 2009.

For example, a hospital is not made for the consultants or more generally for its patients, but for people who go there occasionally, for people who go there for therapy, for relatives, for the people who work there and for all the staff, starting from the cleaners and the ones who do the maintenance, which of course also including the consultants.

A good designer has to think about what the hospital means for all the people who go there. It does not mean the same for people who need care to save their lives, for people who work there or for those who risk getting lost in it. It is always one and the same hospital, but it has to cater for many different people and their needs and requirements. I am not saying that it is easy, but I *am* saying that this is what has to be done.

A few years ago, some students at the Faculty of Architecture in Milan were working on the topic of the airport. I saw their work and felt I had to talk to my friend and colleague about it: I wanted to know why none of the projects had any signs showing entrances and exits, the public side and flight side and so on. His answer was "but we are architects: we don't deal with things like that". I have already pointed out that reality is complex these days. Of course it is not the architect who is responsible for defining active and passive security or the luggage management system, but I am convinced that whoever gives substance to a design must take part in all its phases, first maybe just sitting in and listening, then gradually picking up more and more awareness and the ability to make decisions. Because a hospital could be organised correctly, for example, as an architectural system that identifies flows rather than as a set of specialisations enclosed each in its own silo. The Gallery in the centre of Milan is not just a passageway leading from one square to another: it is a significant place in its own right that also connects fundamental parts of the city, in the process becoming another fundamental part of the city.

What?

Next, you have to ask yourself what the people who will use it will want or have to do with the product.

It is highly probable that the people who use a product an object, place or system) will use it for the purpose for which it was designed. But it is not necessarily so.

To start with, exactly what people do with a product is determined to a certain extent by the product's nature. With a bicycle you can move yourself around, maybe move somebody else or move things. There is not much more you can do with it. But then someone thought of mounting the bicycle on a stand and using the free wheel to turn a grindstone for sharpening knives at home (I'm old enough to have seen this myself). As a result, a generic activity became a specialised one with a twin purpose: movement and activity. It already becomes clear, when we start defining the "who", that every group has different intentions and purposes when using the same product. We can actually say that every product looks different to various categories of people, even though in itself it remains identical.

When it comes to the diversification of functions, recycling becomes an art form when it re-uses cans, bottles, boxes and other things to compose something different. It is an art form, a creative re-use. When you design, you have no idea what your object may mean later in its life, but those who recycle it do: it means getting a new life instead of going to landfill.

THINKING ABOUT IT

For the cleaning staff, a shopping centre has a very different physiognomy from the one that is perceived by or interests a shopkeeper or is perceived by or interests those of us who go there to do our shopping or get new ideas.

A refrigerator is one thing for those of us who use it every day and something quite different for those who have to defrost it or repair it. Yet the object itself remains the same one. The designer has to design all of these facets, like a polyhedron that looks different according to how you turn it.

The question is what activities will be undertaken by the individuals who relate to the products, places or systems. A blender is something that a barman uses for his work, so he wants it to be efficient, safe and always within reach. But a blender is also something that parents use to prepare food for a child (from a very early age), so they want it to be reliable and hygienic, but many only use it sporadically and every time it will be a problem to find the right attachment.

And what about cars? People use them every day in cities, to commute or for work. But on Sundays everyone goes off to the seaside and we'd like it to be different.

The next thing we have to do to enable us to analyse how our products, places and systems will be used is to clarify the various different categories of activities. Because if they are one-off, prevalent or generic they will require different mechanisms for their definition, their analysis and so for finding the right solutions.

The activities carried out (the "what") might be:

- *one-off specialised activities*

The activities that can be carried out with some products are specialised and for specialists.

Some products, places or systems have only one use. A microwave oven's only purpose is to cook or heat food and nothing else (not to dry the cat, as one misguided owner once tried, to her regret). Similarly, a city bus transports people along predetermined and predictable routes.

This makes the "what" easy to define or at least restricts its definition to a very limited area. The purpose of a CAT scan is to help reach a diagnosis (and that is the only thing it can do) in various parts of the body and with a variety of diagnostic possibilities (and that is the only field in which there is any variation).

- *prevalent activities*

The activities that are possible with some products are well defined, but with a broad range of use that does not rule out other possible (and often desirable) activities.

I find that the school building is the example that clarifies this concept best. The purpose of schools is to teach, but they can or should also be a place of some significance for the community. During the school holidays, do we just close them and forget them or do we try to make use of them? One secondary use that has now become quite well established in Italy is that of doubling as polling stations during elections. When we investigate "what" a school building is, we have to manage to identify these aspects, too, regardless of whether or not they may have a bearing on the design.

We all know that railway stations are places passed through by people and goods, but recently they have also become shopping centres. In other words, they are losing their main connotation (travelling) and gaining another of equal importance (as a rendezvous). The same thing is happening to conventional shopping centres, which are increasingly becoming meeting places first and shopping places second. Imagining that the product can fulfil multiple tasks can be an interesting approach, because it enables value to be added to an investment, but it is actually often the consequence of a loss: for example that of the historical town centre as the place where people meet together to exchange things and ideas.

We can also draw a further distinction, between *appropriate* and *inappropriate* uses.

- *Appropriate uses* are the ones that are more or less predictable. To stick with the example of schools, these are uses for polling stations, public meetings or lectures for the elderly, or the school gym may be used for non-scholastic sports activities. In other words, an appropriate use is a predictable but unplanned use that is more or less consistent with the prevailing activity.
- *Inappropriate use*, on the other hand, is anything that might clash with the prevailing activity, such as when the school becomes a refuge for people who have been dislodged by a natural disaster. Another kind of inappropriate use is when a tool is employed for unusual tasks, such as when a fork is used as a corkscrew.

- *generic activities.*

Lastly, there are products, places and systems that have a broad range of usages, such as cutting, writing, connecting and so on. Also in cases such as these, there are various degrees of generic that can spill over into prevailing activities. We can use the scissors that we keep on a workbench or in the kitchen to cut more or less anything, but the scissors we use in the garden are more specialised and the ones we use to prune vines are highly specialised. The same criterion applies to all working tools, for writing and for communicating. A city square should be able to host everyone and also certain specific activities. And what about a scalpel? A tool that was devised for unique, specialised activities, it has become a tool for all generic cutting activities, as everyone with a DIY hobby knows.

How?
Lastly, we have to ask ourselves how the product will be used.

What comes across loud and clear from the definitions provided previously is that the "how" will be determined by the types of activities to be carried out.

If the activity is highly specialised, its use will be guided by more or less rigid protocols. In such cases, you can expect the "who" to be specialists and the "how" to be something that they have had to be taught. Even something as straightforward as driving a car is an activity carried out by specialists, which is what we ourselves are, after we have demonstrated that we have learned to drive and have passed a driving test.

But if an activity is generic, the prevailing use will be based on common experience.

This means that distinctions can also be drawn in this case:

- *use based on protocols*

This is when the use of the product, place or system is determined rigidly by protocols that must be known to the users.

THINKING ABOUT IT

We cannot absolutely rule out the possibility of circumstances where a specialist is not involved (as in the case of an inappropriate use, an accident, indisposition, maintenance and cleaning etc.). In such cases, the system risks becoming mysterious and potentially dangerous for people who are not familiar with it. The best solution would be to make some provision also for these rare cases, for example by blocking certain functions or devising a system capable of regulating itself or of blocking itself to avoid incorrect use being made of it in anomalous circumstances. A good example would be that of firearms.

- *use based on common knowledge*

When the use of a product, place or system is based on common knowledge, it refers to cognitions and abilities that anybody can have learned in the course of training for life. We have to remember, however, that this should not mislead us into thinking that just because we are capable of doing something, everybody else will also be equally capable of doing the same. There are sometimes quite strong differences in habits, knowledge and abilities that depend on our background culture, where we come from, our beliefs, our age and so on.

Talk about "common knowledge" therefore calls for a process of analysis that starts from the "who" and defines geographical and typological areas of diffusion, so as to be able to trigger the right process for defining the "how".

- *use based on instinctive knowledge*

When the use of a product, place or system is based on instinctive knowledge, it refers to the cognitions and abilities that are innate in any human being, such as seeing, grasping, moving and so on.

Yet instinctive knowledge also calls for further definition. There are differences that are well-known and defined, such as differences in ability, which are often related to age (think of the difference between older generations and the ones who were born to information technology), and then there are differences attributable to the reduction in perceptive, sensory and motor capacities brought about by permanent or temporary impairments.

THINKING ABOUT IT

To design something, you have to start from the people, not the things.

It may seem obvious, yet it is not. Here is an example: in what environmental conditions do you watch television at home? If you watch in the dark, you don't have to be a physiologist to know that, even if there is a little ambient light, your eyes will adjust to the strong illumination from the screen. It is as though you were blind to everything except the screen. Would you make a control unit whose recognition calls for excellent eyesight? Never! And yet at least one common radio control unit was originally devised for blind users. Every now and then, the screen tells you to "press the yellow button to record", for example. Or you have to search among the many different keys for the one with the right symbol. This is dreadful design, which reminds us that whoever designed it had no idea that many people have to use tactile qualities instead of colour. He probably thought to himself that "tactile qualities are for blind people, but blind people don't watch television!".

Chapter 3
Looking for the Answer

The need to know whom to ask

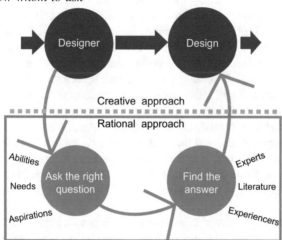

If asking the right question is a part of the design process, looking for the answer is an art.

We are sure that the answer is somewhere out there, but we have to find it.

When I started practising as a professional architect, every architectural studio had its own densely-packed library (as well as the unwieldy great drawings boards!). There were books, magazines and above all catalogues, oceans of catalogues, that were often found to be fatally out of date when you actually needed to consult them. So you would go to your usual trusted supplier to see whether he could dig out the door you wanted, but in Pompeii red. That's what you would do if you were in Milan or some large larger city. But if you were out in the provinces, you would take the train or go to visit a wholesaler, who would then sell you what suited him best.

All that is prehistory now.

These days, everything is on the web and you can find all the information you want, even if you do not live in the throbbing heart of design. That's all very positive, but we have lost the direct contact between demand and production that was one of the driving forces of the unique phenomenon that is Italian design.

© Springer Nature Switzerland AG 2019
L. Bandini Buti, *Ask the Right Question*,
https://doi.org/10.1007/978-3-319-96346-4_3

THINKING ABOUT IT

The sixties and seventies were interesting years when Italy developed and disseminated design. Many architects started working in design because the market had nothing to offer that suited the architecture they were creating. In Milan, for example, there was Azucena,[1] which started operations in 1947 because a group of young Milanese architects and businessmen decided there was a market for furniture that some of them would design and the others would produce, a repertoire of furnishings ready for the homes they were designing at the time. Azucena gave them a hand to make them and then put them in its catalogue. The approach adopted was not structured, but it provided an opening for one man's needs to become another man's excellence.

One thing was certain: at that time, nobody had yet woken up to the fact that good design was and could also become good business.

The days are long gone when a designer could think he was capable of understanding everything (doubling as a technician, a psychologist, a sociologist, a doctor and more besides) and that all he had to do was read things up in books and magazines. Today's culture is a culture of complexities. Even a car is not just a simple self-propelling vehicle (remember the old days, when it was enough if it moved?): these days it is an object that has become a fully integrated part of everyone's lives, offering high performance, comfort and safety and conveying a lot of meaning about each individual's status.

A smattering of several disciplines is not enough any more: you need to activate the ability to involve them in their entirety, and others too. That is what makes the specialised "ask the right question" tool so necessary, since it provides the questions about man, the environment and systems. Which now brings us to the need to look for the answers to those questions.

***

Finding the right answer to each question is not so obvious an issue. It is not a matter of interviewing people or of digging deep into the designer's knowledge, but of finding the answer in a vast ocean of written or computerised information or in the knowledge of informed individuals. The purpose of "finding the answer" is not to serve up precooked solutions, but to find those (organisations or people) who deal with accessibility for all and navigating in the great sea of objective data (manuals, laws etc.).

The challenge today in the internet is not to hope that the data will be there, but how to find them. Looking for the answer becomes doubling as a search engine about accessible design and enabling the question to be focused in the right place.

While the main place to search for the right answer is in the world of information in general, an enormous influence is exerted by the examples given by good practices. Actually seeing bathroom fittings, touching handles and turning taps can be a lot more rewarding than reading a whole host of descriptions.

---

[1]Azucena is an Milanese firm that started operations in 1947, producing works of design to cater for the needs of a group of (then young) designers: Luigi Caccia Dominioni, Corrado Corradi Dell'Acqua, Ignazio Gardella and Maria Teresa and Franca Tosi.

THINKING ABOUT IT

If we remember that a design is the result of a value chain, it is clear that all the stakeholders in the design process—the decision-makers, designers, executors, managers and users—must be able to have their say consciously, although they probably do not have any specific tools for doing so. The kind of tools I mean are the ones that an engineer, an architect or a designer might wield for his profession: all those people who know how to read a technical drawing, for example. The end user will almost certainly not be familiar with the abstraction of how things are represented, but there is also no guarantee that a specialist in a non-design discipline will be any the wiser.

Yet we all have the ability to analyse the reality around us, especially if we experience it ourselves. And what could be better than direct experience?

Direct experience—seeing, touching and using—does not call for the ability to interpret anything, unlike what happens in the case of designs or images. It would be the best tool for applying interdisciplinarity, but it is difficult to achieve, primarily for practical reasons. You have to know where to go and why you are going there; you then have to reach the place and then ask to be able to interact with the things you find there. If you go into a showroom, you will probably not have many difficulties, but if you have to go to a public or private venue or, even worse, into a private home, you certainly cannot take accessibility for granted.

I'd like to see someone organise a census of good practices and create an organisation to manage visits in which people could touch accessibility solutions "with their hands". For example, there may be bathrooms that are absolutely compliant with the standards set by the law and with good practices, but that also look great.

Design for All reminds us that it is better to be "realistic and do things" than "theoretical and not do anything".

Reality on the ground is often very different from scientific/academic models. When you work for manufacturers, there are often no real times and resources for conducting accurate or scientifically correct research. For example, it is very hard to convince an auto manufacturer that he should invest money and six months of time to obtain statistically significant data about the appraisal of the knob on a gear lever. It should also be remembered that such needs are nearly always only revealed during the actual design process and there really is no time to put everything on hold. It is so tempting just to give up: it is the easiest solution.

THINKING ABOUT IT

More than 20 years ago, I happened to have to evaluate the correct qualities of how the hand would grip a device located behind the steering wheel of a car (a steering column switch) that was substantially bulkier than the ones on the market at the time. I needed to have anthropometric data about the hand (the distance to push and the distance to pull) that were not available in any manual of anthropometrics.

But I had to come up with an answer in 15 days. That was what the programmes told me.

We obviously could not organise a widespread research project about anthropometric data in just fifteen days, but we could conduct an honest survey of some fifty individuals chosen more because they were prepared to do it than because of their statistical significance. We were creatives and we thought of collecting data about as many individuals as possible (by asking them to make a photocopy of their hands!), so that we could appraise the statistical distribution of the data sought in relation to data used in the manual of anthropometrics: the length of the hand. What we found was that the ratio between the length of the hand and the data we sought was $0.68 \pm 0.02\%$ in all individuals (both male and female). To the utter horror of the scientists, we then deduced that, if we multiplied the lengths of the hands in all the manuals by these values, we would get the data we needed. Of course we could not lay claim to any scientific certainty, but to a good approximation and, above all, in time.

***

I already said that finding the answers is an art. It may actually be anything but straightforward, since you have to be able to distinguish between "what really is" and "the idea of things" that individuals have. If you want to know the propensity for change of an individual who goes home with a new, full-blown pathology, you have to ask questions pertinent to the case. The answers we dug out were certainly related more to his hopes than to reality. We repeated them both to his doctor and to the members of his family who lived with him and found three different versions, on which we then built a model that may not have been strictly true, but was certainly the most probable. We also derived some important information that had not been expressed in so many words, nor even asked for, about how willing the individual was to tackle his new condition.

3.1   Finding the Right Help

Every right question must be addressed to the right interviewee and in the right ways.

It's no straightforward challenge: a designer's common sense or common knowledge are not enough to be able to tackle this task appropriately. That is why you need to access specialised information.

THINKING ABOUT IT

We are often tempted to put our trust in nothing but "common sense". But "common sense" alone is not enough: you have to give your thinking an organised structure. By this I don't mean that you can do without common sense, but that it is not sufficient. In a friendly diatribe with the late Isao Hosoe,[2] he maintained that common sense was sufficient and there was no need to invent new disciplines, illustrating his argument with the fact that peasants had always made perfect tools for themselves, long before such a thing as ergonomics existed. But I pointed out that the peasant was at one and the same time the designer, manufacturer and user of his tools. He enshrined interdisciplinarity in himself. The product catered perfectly for him, for his needs and for the environment. These days,

---

[2]Isao Hosoe (Tokyo, 8 March 1942–Milan, 3 October 2015) was a Japanese engineer and designer who moved to Milan in 1967 to work with Gio Ponti and Alberto Rosselli, before opening his own prestigious professional practice.

those who design are not the end users any more, but may actually be very far away from them, so have to acquire tools to learn about needs.

"Finding the answer" does not mean chatting with your friends in a café.

On what sources can you draw to find the answers, and what resources can you use?

The sources are primarily all the people who will use the end product or come into contact with it in one way or another; then there are the experts who know how to investigate humanity, the experts of design and the specialised technicians who know how to investigate objects and the associations that bring together the various categories of people who are disadvantaged in one way or another and protect them and their interests.

(A) Sources

- *Individuals*

The richest source of original information is that of the individuals who will interact with the artefact. There is a very articulated range of survey methods available for investigating subjective information, which should be chosen on the basis of the kind of results you expect and the times and resources you have at your disposal.

There are many tried and tested methods of data collection. Italian standard UNI 11377 (Usability of industrial products) furnishes a list of tools for collecting subjective data—interviews, questionnaires, expert assessments, contextual observation of users and/or ethnographic groups, task analysis, focus groups, thinking aloud and sensory quality assessment (Sequam)—which it describes in detail.

UNI 11377 Standard—Usability of Industrial Products

The most important methods used for collecting subjective data are listed in Italy's UNI 11377 standard (Usability of industrial products, Part 2: Methods and tools, September 2010).

– *interviews.*

The interview is certainly the indirect and qualitative investigation tool most commonly used in the psychosocial sciences. It is a very versatile knowledge-gathering instrument, well suited to capturing the dimension of subjectivity, without prejudice to the attention that has to be paid to the more objective phenomena to be investigated.

– *questionnaires.*

This tool uses a checklist to enable users to express their opinions. Objective issues can be investigated effectively in this way.

– *expert assessments.*

These are based on the expert's skills and knowledge.

– *contextual observation of users and/or ethnographic groups.*

The observation of ethnographic groups is a technique derived from anthropology that aims to extrapolate the greatest amount of information possible about people's lifestyles by observing their behaviour without interfering with them.

– *task analysis.*

This entails analysing the tasks related to the expected use to be made of the product.

– *focus groups.*

This is a method of investigation that is based on involving multiple users at the same time, in a sort of collective interview that takes place in a group of 6–8 people.

– *thinking aloud,*

This is an empirical methodology that invites users to express their thoughts and comments out loud to accompany their actions as they interact with the object being tested. In practice, users are asked to fulfil a given task, while expressing their sensations, opinions and/or frustrations out loud.

– *sensory quality assessment* (*Sequam*).

This comprises analysing subjective sensations related to the sensory qualities conveyed by the object when it comes into contact with man.

• *The experts*

In many cases, the nature of the question calls for detailed answers, sometimes with a very high degree of specialisation. For example, if the issue under discussion is the possibility that a car driver will be distracted by information overload, we have to ask how the information can be expressed correctly and what technologies can be used to achieve this aim. To answer this, we need to talk to experts in health, of the mind, of perception and of mobility: these are professionals who tend to have a high level of specialisation and who are capable of furnishing the right answers to the "right questions" we have formulated.

THINKING ABOUT IT

What happens in an operating theatre can be described well in literature and you can also ask the people who work there, but you certainly need to obtain some very advanced expert information if you want to know how emergencies are managed, for example, or how the hierarchy functions. Similarly, when your task is to adapt a home to suit the needs of a specific individual with specific disabilities, it is vital to be able to ask expert doctors about how that individual's impairments are likely to evolve, so as to ensure that you will be making the home good for today, but also for the future.

One and the same question can be addressed to multiple sources: it will be the nature of the question and its degree of complexity that will suggest how many and which sources you should address.

What characteristics do these experts have? Here is a rudimentary SWOT analysis:

- *Strengths*
  Experts are professionals who have developed expertise that can be recognised as useful, necessary or indispensable at a certain stage of development of the design process.
- *Weaknesses*
  Experts should not be expected to have a global view of issues: that is not their task.
- *Opportunities*
  You have to know how to formulate the right question, which calls for you to understand what part of their knowledge you need for the issue at stake. For example, you can show them a range of handles and ask them which one could be suitable for a specific pathology and why. Or which colours can be distinguished by a certain category of colour-blind people.
- *Threats*
  Make sure that the experts operate in their own field of expertise and do not invade any others. A health expert must confirm whether there is an issue of the perception of obstacles that calls for attention to be paid to the environment, for example: his task is not to insist that the environment should be white!

- ***Designers***

Designers are experts in the design process in the broadest sense of the term (designing, executing and managing).

Of all the people who take part in the working group, the designer is one with specific characteristics and responsibilities. He is the one who must first listen to opinions, collect and sort data and explore the contradictory issues that come to light, then make the ultimate decisions: once he has decided for steel, reinforced concrete, wood and so on, there is no going back on his decision, except for the possibility of adaptation that he himself inserts into the design.

The design process is intrinsically complex and potentially difficult to execute. Yet we have to remember that, in everyday practice and the more straightforward of projects (in terms of their nature or of the technology involved), a good professional who is trained to apply the principles of Design for All may work autonomously and need only draw on additional information, which may be informal in nature, from a variety of sources. In other words, he can benefit from what he has learned from a suitably Design for All-oriented training.

This will happen when universities realise that these approaches and tools have what it takes to be the necessary support for advanced design work, which makes it worthwhile including them in their study curricula!

What characteristics do designers have? Again, from a SWOT:

- *Strengths*
  Designers who are specialised in DfA have acquired the ability to see the complexity of the issues at stake, including aspects of how systems are managed, and are vital members of the working group. The working group is the ideal theoretical condition for tackling what is inevitably always a complex design challenge, such as that of active ageing.
- *Weaknesses*
  There are designers (many) who pay attention to the issues of form and others who focus on energy challenges or on the profitability of each operation. Very often, however, they may be rather insensitive to the need to cater for humanity, for all humanity with its needs and requirements, or they do not want to work that way, or are incapable of doing so. They are often afraid that their creative wings will be clipped!
- *Opportunities*
  DfA designers are designers who have developed specific knowledge and techniques.
  Decision-makers who want to create products that "cater for all" must employ this kind of designer. The fact is that the choice of designer impacts fatally on the final result. Unlike what is often mistakenly believed, the DfA approach favours creative innovation because, by focusing on the individual, it launches new challenges that call for new solutions in terms both of utility and of form.
- *Threats*
  The risk is that often complex and costly methodologies may be applied acritically. If you have to redesign a family's bathroom for grandad who has had an operation, is it possible and realistic to conduct a complex, costly project? Usually no! So there is a series of levels of approach to use, remembering that it is better to be "realistic and do things" than "theoretical and not do anything".

THINKING ABOUT IT

When we say that a DfA project has to involve the entire value chain, we are talking about the fact that its nature is already determined from the moment when the designer receives the commission. I was once asked to work on a series of editorial offices, where I had to put expensive patches over the work of the archistar who had solved the architectural issues (brilliantly), but created acoustically unsustainable situations in the process. For him, human beings just got in the way of his designs. If the top decision-makers had been aware of DfA, they could have made provision for these inconveniences and tackled them consciously, rather than having to deal with them after the event. That is why I say that DfA should be taught in schools of management and not only in faculties of architecture.

- *Specialised technicians*

These are building, product or system technicians who are specialised in specific sectors (structures, plant, applied information technology, management, furnishings, accessories, materials, legislation, orientation etc.).

What characteristics do specialised technicians have?

- *Strengths*
  If specialised technicians have had a DfA training they will be capable of providing solutions to unusual or complex issues, imagining creative solutions and not just trusting in good practice or the way things have always been done before. For example, they may think of flexible hydraulic systems that would enable substantial alterations to be made in bathrooms in future, without having to invest in expensive building work.
- *Weaknesses*
  These specialists risk having a strong bias in favour of hands-on applications and so very little propensity for dialogue and innovation (inventiveness).

THINKING ABOUT IT

Specialists are often so focused on their own discipline that they have difficulty thinking inclusively. I once suggested my idea to a major archaeological site of classifying its visitors on the basis of three categories I had identified: the ones who want to see the essentials, the ones who want "their hand to be held" and the ones who already know but want to learn more. They told me I was right. But when I asked which of the monuments were of the "must see" category, they told me that they were all "must see". That's because every rock is quite rightly of great value to an archaeologist. So of course the project never took off! In addition, I did not even manage to persuade them to tell me the dates of the monuments, because it is a matter of controversy between the various schools of thought, so the best thing is not to say anything at all. That is what happens when the management is very specialised. It would not happen if the managers took care of conservation, but also of usability. But the mere idea was apparently scandalous! So I find myself wondering whether it would be better for a large car manufacturer to be run by someone who knows how to make cars, or someone who knows how to have them made, but also how to sell them?

- ## *The associations*

There is another major category of bodies that are inexhaustible sources of information, often with considerable detail. These are the associations that deal with particular categories of individuals who have specific impairments: associations of blind people, of people with celiac disease, of paraplegics and many others.

What characteristics do specialised associations have?

- *Strengths*
  These associations are very expert in their areas of competence; they nurture institutional relations with public and private bodies and with the system of legislation and standards. They maintain active relations with many individuals and their families.

- *Weaknesses*
  Since these associations are very specialised and vigorously oriented, they are generally extremely short-sighted about any forms of impairment other than the ones that they themselves represent.
- *Opportunities*
  These associations should be used for what they are capable of offering, which is never the DfA project of proposing benefits for everyone while also solving the issues of interest to their specific categories.

(B) Resources

What resources can we use to access these sources? One typical trait of the present day is a proliferation of such resources. So where do we go to find the right help? The first thing we turn to is the web, which we consult every day; then there is printed matter – books and magazines, in their hardcopy form or as the increasingly widespread PDF. In fact, the difference between the various resources lies more in how they process and present information than in the nature of the support, except for the ease of access to them.

> THINKING ABOUT IT
>
> Our media culture ensures us that the information is all out there somewhere: we just have to find it. We even reach the paradox that many students are so sure that everything is on the web that they have lost the ability to criticise and have replaced reflection and the search for a solution with the ability to surf the web. And that sounds the death knell for creativity. Yet it is also true that surfing the web is an art that entails orienting your search and above all knowing how to discern good information from bad. The major difference between the web and the printed page is that the web is the product of a widespread, anonymous community, while a printed work has had the go-ahead from a publisher, who stands warranty for it but also acts as a selector of the information it contains.

- **Websites**

With the Internet, we are submerged under a flood of information.

These days, the institutions have an official web presence through which they converse with us: some of them actually use nothing but the web. So you have to know how to surf if you want to find the right information: analyses, proposals and solutions for certain situation, which may be very specific, and information about how to adapt places, products and systems.

What characteristics does web-based information have?

- *Strengths*
  We are reasonably certain that we will find the information we are looking for in the great sea of the web: the problem is how to get to it.
- *Weaknesses*
  Not all information in the web is reliable: you have to be careful not to fall into the easy snares laid by advertising or the traps of superficial sloppiness.
  A great many websites are hosted by associations or other authorities: in this case, you have to avoid the tendency to focus on a specific disability and not on

how it connects to the context. There are still very few sites that really discuss Design for All, while a great many of them tackle issues related to particular aspects or pathologies.

- *Opportunities*
  You have to know how to use keywords for running a web search, not only in your own language, but preferably also in English, since that gives you access to international sites. The keywords may be related to the method of the approach (Design for All of course, but also Inclusive design, Ergonomics, Usability, Human factors, accessibility etc.), to a certain pathology (disability, visual impairment, blind, colour blindness, celiac etc.), to places and activities (bathroom, kitchen, housework, sleeping etc.) or to products (wheelchair, rollator, crutches, artificial limbs, technical aids, stairlifts etc.).

- ***Hardcopy and online magazines***

Magazines are more or less targeted containers of information and examples (often illustrated with drawings and photographs). Hardcopy and online magazines together constitute a clear conceptual category, since they are relevant to the here-and-now and can zoom into focus on very specific sectors.

What characteristics do magazines have?

- *Strengths*
  Magazines are a great tool for collecting examples of good solutions. They typically deal with clearly-defined fields of issues, target specific readers and suggest specialised solutions also through the industry advertising they carry. The information they contain is not only about what has already happened, but also about what is happening as they are published. Many of them offer stimuli about aesthetic trends in design that can help achieve the principle that states "if it is not attractive, it is not Design for All".
- *Weaknesses*
  Very few of them deal with issues related to Design for All and/or active ageing.
- *Opportunities*
  All the magazines that deal with ergonomics, Design for All and other design disciplines, as well as the ones that deal with evident cases of impairments, may contain useful information.
  Useful information can sometimes also be found in publications with no specific orientation, such as magazines covering the latest developments in architecture and design, which may direct their readers towards the latest new trends, or in magazines that specialise in certain fields of goods (floor products, doors and windows etc.) or types of goods (for the kitchen, the bathroom, homes in the countryside etc.).
- *Threats*
  Magazines are very much influenced by their advertisers, which means that they may not be very reliable.

- ***Hardcopy and online books***

Regardless of whether they are hardcopy or in an e-format, books should always be treated as a specific conceptual category: they are linked to how culture develops, are preserved as time goes by (constituting our historical memory) and are authoritative. The fact that all the most important reference books (from the Bible onwards) have always been hardcopy has even led people here in Italy to coin a proverb to say that a well-grounded person "speaks like a printed book".

While much of our research starts these days on the Internet, we also make ample use of libraries, especially university libraries. Printed books can be found in specialised bookshops, also on the web.

What characteristics do books have?

- *Strengths*
  Books are authoritative because the technology used to produce them calls for technological investment, which requires careful selection on the part of publishers. This is a guarantee of their commitment, but not necessarily of quality.
- *Weaknesses*
  More and more self-published books are coming out and the trend is destined to increase: their only guarantee is the author's own authority. Meanwhile, new technologies (digital printing and the web) are breaking down publishers' monopolies and creating space for potentially very interesting niche products.
- *Opportunities*
  There are books, some of them very authoritative, that deal with the issues of Design for All, accessibility or design in general. Then there are also books that are made up mostly of illustrations (a little like magazines), although they are nearly always carefully selected and broader in range.

  Another to some extent exclusive category of books is the kind that publish the proceedings of conferences and congresses, which often contain very specific and often unprecedented, up-to-the-minute information and forecasts. Some publishers specialise in these, listing many conference and congress proceedings in their catalogues.

  Printed books also leave space for other forms of communication. These may be in the form of text but interactive or available as a PDF, which means that they are not interactive, but have the advantage of being easy for people with sight impairments to read and allow voice synthesis for blind people.

  Graduation theses are an often unexplored terrain, although it is one that may be packed with stimuli and original information. The only guarantees that the thesis is serious are the reputation of the university and of the tutor. But it may be difficult to come across them.

3.2 Finding the Right Things

Buying consciously—right and attractive

When you set out to develop a virtuous design, you have to be able to source the market for materials, products, objects or systems that will enable you to create it. But if the sanitary fittings for all that everyone designs are always white and look as though they belong in a hospital, it will be very hard to imagine suitable bathrooms that are also attractive. So what the market has to offer is decisive for a good design. It is no coincidence that DfA states that a good design is the result of the entire value chain.

THINKING ABOUT IT

Ever since the 1970s, ergonomics has successfully tackled issues of the harm that lurks in the industrial workplace, proposing alterations and solutions for factories. But when the focus shifted from the factory to the office, we realised that we could not solve things case by case: the production of the objects, furnishings and equipment used in offices had to be redirected towards the requirements of an environmentally correct design process. That is how ergonomics started studying design and that is how furniture started being made that was suitable for the changing ways we work, in the process also quite rightly creating good business.

Here's an example: a firm that produces equipment for playgrounds has promised to include multisensory inclusive items in its catalogue. Wonderful. But the question is: will the buyers (local councils, hotels, organisations, schools, tourist resorts etc.) be aware enough to introduce these virtuous games, or will they languish in the catalogues? Of course we need conscientious manufacturers with good catalogues, but we also have to raise awareness among the decision-makers who use the catalogues.

If it is true that designing and creating objects requires the use of materials, furnishings and equipment produced and made available by third parties, then inclusive design oriented to cater for people's—all people's!—real needs calls for consciously good products.

It is certainly a complex art to choose between the enormous range of products on offer today, between their much-boasted, amazing capabilities and their more or less true promises. Asking the right question enables us to get to know who our users are, what characteristics and needs they have, since these days we need to have suitable parameters for interpreting what is available to us.

(A) Knowledge

The first thing we need is to get to know what everyone needs, in particular when those needs are special, a situation that puts people at a potential disadvantage.

THINKING ABOUT IT

In the practical research conducted by my group to identify everyone's needs in the course of the work commissioned by our clients, we have often used people with difficulties as amplifiers of the issues associated with usability. When we studied how people interface with the domestic oven, we used pregnant women, women with small children, people with poor hand grips and cognitive difficulties, not so as to make an oven for everyone, but to get some decisive answers. If you ask perfectly healthy twenty-somethings if they have any difficulties controlling the food they are cooking, they will not even know what you are talking about. Try asking a new mum with a baby in her arms!

This might induce us to consider what solutions are most suitable for the needs thus discovered and find which product available on the market (which must also avoid singling out and labelling its users as people with disabilities and actually be attractive) caters for these requirements. Very often, we shall find that there is actually nothing that quite fits the bill, so we have to choose the best possible compromise.

What characteristics do the right things have?

- *Strengths*
  The "right questions" provide designers with tools that certainly help them source the right products.
- *Weaknesses*
  It may be difficult to distinguish between a product's real characteristics and the ones promised by advertising.
- *Opportunities*
  When you need to find out what is available, you look for firms that supply products for all, or at least products that can be used correctly. So you consult catalogues, showrooms, exhibitions and trade fairs.
  To help you find your way there are organisations and other bodies that see nothing themselves, but have acted on your behalf to classify the firms that cater for specific criteria. In practice, they are specialised search engines that can be found on the Internet.
  But care must be paid, as images alone may be misleading. Specialised photographers are very good at manipulating images!

(B) What Is Available: The Right Supply

A correct level of knowledge enables you to analyse what is available with an eye on the qualities concerned with an inclusive design approach.

The first step in choosing the right range of products available is to acquire the certainty that comes when the products are furnished with a guarantee, such as the Design for All Quality Label,[3] whose serious approach and credibility certify and guarantee their subject matter.

Products recommended by authorities that deal with specific pathologies are also very reliable, although with the proviso that they nearly always tend to be highly reminiscent of hospital equipment and rather inflexible in use. In other words, the model adopted by these authorities is a specific pathology at the greatest extent of its disabling impact: this they then set up in opposition to the rest of the world, which they consider fundamentally to be privileged.

---

[3]The Design for All Quality Label was established in 2009 by the association Design for All Italia to certify the DfA characteristics of products, places and systems.

Although specialised literature contains illustrations and descriptions of good practices that describe how correct products and solutions can be adopted, the most important source remains a search among all the products available on the market, analysing them through the lens of an approach for All.

THINKING ABOUT IT

Autogrill received the Design for All Quality Label for its Villoresi Est motorway service area structure just outside Milan. But the architectural staff pointed out to me that their core business was catering and they were also very good at designing structures, although they were less good at subtler assessments of furnishings and accessories. When they had to choose a chair, a table or cutlery, they felt that did not have suitable tools for making decisions based on DfA. They said that they would welcome the spread of such quality certification, because it would give them more certainty.

What characteristics does the right supply have?

- *Strengths*
  The market almost certainly offers products that may cater for the requirements found to feature in a given design. There are also firms that specialise in offering products adapted to suit people with particular needs.
- *Weaknesses*
  An accurate assessment may not be very straightforward when all that you have to go by is photographs and it is hard to access the product itself.
- *Threats*
  A designer or architect may often want to take the easiest way out by sticking acritically to what he has always done before (for example by choosing sanitary fittings and bathroom accessories that look as though they came straight out of a hospital, because that way he is sure that the authorities will raise no objections). But common sense would adopt a very different position.

3.3 Finding the Right Examples

Good practices

As I mentioned earlier, you do not have to have any specialised tools or knowledge to have a direct, hand-on relationship with things: the approach is intrinsically interdisciplinary.

Many people who act as links in the value chain almost certainly have no such specialised tools for giving meaning to what is represented in technical drawings or images. Ultimately, it is so much better to see, touch and try out real situations and maybe discuss them with people who use them every day!

To find the right examples, you have to be able to consult good practices and try to make them accessible. Just imagine how interesting it would be to visit a mul-tipurpose classroom in a school, a bathroom that is not for people with disabilities, but really suitable for everyone, hotel rooms that are both accessible and excellent and so on, getting direct, hands-on feedback about the pros and cons experienced by people using them.

Good DfA practices in architecture are virtuous projects in relation to which we are sometimes aware of the names of the architects, of the clients who commissioned them, of their aims and needs, of the costs involved, the difficulties encountered and the results achieved.

Good practices may encompass an entire system (a house, a retirement home for the elderly, the lobby and public areas in a hotel etc.), or equally well just certain details (a system of doors, shelves suitable for everyone and so on), culminating in the correct usage of an individual product (a non-slip floor, interactive signage etc.). If you are a designer, good practices can provide an efficient means for communicating the possible results of what you want to achieve to your client.

The possibility of visiting the right example is certainly a complex issue. There are questions about how to discover and guarantee it, then issues of privacy that may be comparable to the ones encountered when accessing historical buildings that are not open to the general public. I believe that this kind of activity should be organised by an authority that offers a guarantee, such as a foundation, a cultural body, a university or some other public authority.

- *Visitable examples*

These are functioning places that can be visited. They may be any kind of built environment, such as houses, flats, hotel rooms, classrooms, meeting rooms, city spaces, children's playgrounds and so on. We need to try to classify the kinds of places that might constitute examples of good practices, either as a whole or at least in terms of certain aspects, drawing up a documentary record of the degree to which they can be visited and everything else necessary.

THINKING ABOUT IT

The difficult thing about acquiring tangible experience with real places is reflected in the difficulty encountered by people whose work involves rehabilitation, giving their patients the opportunity to try and test real places that are different from the ones they were accustomed to frequenting before the event that led to their acquiring a disability. To go some way towards overcoming this difficulty, standard sample places have been created where patients can undergo rehabilitation in using their homes. This is a good practice that deserves to be more widespread, among other things because it conveys an understanding that an adapted home cannot be a "hospital home" that the individual and above all those who live with him would find ugly and alienating. In other words, it ought to be a DfA house.[4]

What characteristics do visitable examples have?

- *Strengths*
  You can get to know them directly.

---

[4]One example is the experimental residential unit known as the *Casa Agevole*, designed by the architect Fabrizio Vescovo and built in 2004 by the Santa Lucia Foundation, which created a full-scale model on its own premises in Rome.

You can source their addresses from the social services, hospitals or other channels, such as social networks. You can collect documentation and images about them, or technical data (drawings, specifications, lists of suppliers).

- *Weaknesses*
  It may sometimes be difficult or inopportune to visit them.
- *Opportunities*
  You can gather direct information about the pros and cons and collect the subjective opinions of the people who manage and/or use them.

- ***Other examples***

It may not always be reasonable to visit some examples of excellent buildings and places, maybe because they are geographically remote or because they have been transformed or have become outdated. Nevertheless, many are or have been active locations even if they cannot now be visited, which means that familiarity with them may be a rich source of ideas and experiences.

In the first place, you have to unearth the sources capable of supplying information about good practices, regardless of their geographical location. You can then find documentary evidence about the building's structural aspects, together with the perceptive, sensory and social reactions to them deriving from how it has really been used in practice.

What characteristics do examples in general have?

- *Strengths*
  When you can draw on an extensive range of examples, you have a greater chance of finding some that are truly excellent. For example, things that have taken place in other countries and that may be in compliance with different and more advanced legislation.
- *Weaknesses*
  You cannot visit them, so you cannot get direct experience of them (it is difficult to get a true perception of the built environment, which is more than what you see), nor can you investigate the experience of the people who use them.
- *Opportunities*
  The sources you use may also be magazines, websites, social networks etc., with representations of built environments places that you can only experience through images and written descriptions.
- *Threats*
  You may find yourself being influenced more by the journalist who wrote the article than by the architect who designed the environment.

- ***Designs***

Another source comes from unexecuted designs, which cannot be verified in the flesh, but have the advantage of tending to be innovative. They are the results of competitions or graduation theses and are usually interesting, even though they have not—or not yet—been built. You have to be capable of making a critical analysis of the examples selected, so as to highlight the aspects that come across as good practices.

What characteristics do the right designs have?

- *Strengths*
  They are easily likely to be innovative and in some cases may be very much so (as in the case of competitions or graduation theses).
- *Weaknesses*
  No check has ever been run on just how feasible they really are, in terms of both construction and use.
- *Opportunities*
  They may come from anywhere in the world, so offer a broad perspective of the state of the art.

- ***Documentation***

Another vital source of information is the relevant literature, covering what has been written about the issue in question.

At one time, a literature search was a long and laborious process, because you had to know how to find your way around libraries, with filing systems, cross-references and more. These days, the web has made such searches available to everybody and it is densely packed with information. Researchers have developed a specific ability to surf this immense sea that contains everything and its opposite, yet to do so effectively they must also have learned the far less easy skill of how to identify the most useful keywords.

Managing to attribute the correct significance to the information you find in the web has also become a really specialised skill, involving the ability to distinguish between reliable information and promotions or advertising.

When you are familiar with the literature, it enables you to keep up with the state of the art, its developments and its prospects, so to place your own intended design work in a context of history and space.

In the case of the right examples that you come across in the literature, you have to ensure that the data you collect does not consist of photographs alone, but also includes relief or executive drawings and descriptions of the characteristics of the products or building works in question. This will then enable you to shape a clear idea of the characteristics of the finished work and make some targeted deductions to use in your own operations.

What characteristics does documentation have?

- *Strengths*
  Compilations of documentation can be useful and sometimes indispensable for using good practices to source great ideas for the design you are working on.
- *Weaknesses*
  Technical documentation is very often unavailable or insufficiently detailed.

- *Opportunities*
  When you collect documentation, you have to search for all the data that can be useful for pursuing your research. Once you have identified an interesting example, you can use references to develop your research further, for example starting from the geographical location, from the architect or from his client, to seek and find further technical data and information about how the project was managed.

3.4 Finding the Right Data

Data are not everything, but they go a long way

Have you ever come across a bathroom for people with disabilities, complete with all the accessories, a higher-than-usual toilet, handles, grab bars and all the other contraptions… but down in a basement without a lift? I have! Someone insisted that there should be a bathroom for people with disabilities that complied with the standards, then checked its compliance… but it was not his job to check whether anyone could actually reach it.

And have you ever seen lifts that are a great boon for people using wheelchairs who have to change level in a building… but end up being used by others to store garbage until collection day comes around? In that case, nobody can say that full accessibility has been denied: it's guaranteed, of course, but what is denied is the human dignity of those who are expected to share the lift with the garbage, because a person with a disability is not a second-class citizen.[5]

No design can ignore the need to comply with the law and the application of standards, both because the law is binding and because it constitutes what ought to be the minimum standard in a civilised country. Yet the problem is that these supposedly minimum standards nearly always end up doubling as maximum standards, so in practice run the risk of becoming severe restrictions: they wash consciences clean and avoid the need for designers to think about the issues at stake.

This is where we need to draw a distinction between the concepts of description and prescription. Description means that we ask for accessibility in the way we consider to be most opportune and suitable, while prescription is made up of numerical values that are easy to tick off on a checklist. A description is of course open to interpretation and I'm afraid it may not be suitable for a population of dreamers, voyagers and smart alecs, as the proverb says that we Italians are. But I shall take this line of reasoning no further, as it might lead me off topic.

---

[5]This brings a little anecdote to mind. When one of the editions of the Triennale was inaugurated, Italy's Prime Minister of the day, Giovanni Spadolini (a great man, but also quite a big one), ended up wedged into the armchair provided for the press conference. This caused quite a stir among his young staff, who had to change the armchairs in all the subsequent events.

Domestic and international legislation has been tackling the issue of disability since the 1950s, when the barrier-free movement in the United States started responding to the needs of veterans with disabilities, pushing for changes in social policy and design practices to abolish physical barriers. The first accessibility standard (*Making Buildings Accessible to and Usable by the Physically Handicapped*) was issued in 1961.

- ### *Standards and laws*

Standards are indications and guidelines for good practice (which only become cogent if they are bolstered by the law), while the law expects compliance. This applies to domestic laws governing accessibility and the means whereby they are administered, together with laws that transpose European Directives and UNI, CEN and ISO standards governing accessibility.

What characteristics do standards and laws have?

- *Strengths*
  Nearly everything is covered by standards. The existence of obligatory laws guarantees that certain basic steps will be taken. Without the laws that make them obligatory, accessible toilets, ramps and kerb cuts would be a great rarity.
- *Weaknesses*
  Compliance with standards does not always translate into catering for real needs, because standards deal with everything that can be measured, but not with human dignity and often also not with common sense. Standards deal with ensuring that certain steps are taken, not with how taking them is managed. Standards are often applied to individual objects and not to the system as a whole (e.g. compliant toilets in inaccessible rooms).
- *Threats*
  Literal compliance with standards and laws is often no more than an alibi, because it furnishes designers with the facile illusion that they have done everything necessary.

- ### *Tools*

A good design calls for data to be collected, interpreted and translated into the steps in the design process.

Many disciplines have taken steps to elaborate design and analysis methodologies and to provide tools for collecting data and elaborating them correctly. Leading the field, Design for All offers methods for designing for everyone based on an holistic approach, overcoming the concept of specialised designs for people with disabilities.

Other discipline that also tackle issues related to the usability of products, places and systems and/or to disability include ergonomics, human factors design, inclusive design and universal design.

What characteristics do tools for collecting data and subjective impressions have?

- *Strengths*
  The tools that have been elaborated for investigating subjective impressions and collecting data have been verified and are effective.
- *Weaknesses*
  Generally speaking, these tools are disproportionate and too expensive for simple design undertakings.
- *Opportunities*
  There are many different kinds of tools and methods that can be used for inclusive design processes: expert assessments, task analysis, user testing, contextual observation of users and/or ethnic groups, questionnaires, interviews, focus groups and co-design methods (workshops with users).

- ***Manuals***

There are many manuals that can be used for inclusive design processes: manuals about Design for All and ergonomics, manuals of anthropometrics, specific accessibility manuals and manuals about individual pathologies. But manuals in themselves do not solve all the issues related to searching for solutions. While it is true that they provide an important support to the design process, it is also true that they are tools that only enable designers to contemplate the physical aspects of places and situations, not individuals' perceptive, cognitive and personal experiential issues.

Once this has been established, the important role played by manuals in the design process deserves recognition.

What characteristics do manuals have?

- *Strengths*
  Manuals provide information, such as anthropometric data, that might otherwise be quite difficult to source: they furnish practical solutions to problems, tending to make them easy to apply. Manuals are a good starting point for a design process.
- *Weaknesses*
  Manuals have to be generic, referring to the standard cases that are encountered most frequently. The data they provide have to be interpreted, to adapt them to individual situations. Manuals should never be treated acritically, as though they offered pre-packaged solutions.
- *Threats*
  There is a risk that people will think that the data supplied by a manual are always right and exhaustive, also for specific individuals and/or situations.

THINKING ABOUT IT

Many people think that manuals are all you need to get a design right.

But manuals focus on people who are healthy and efficient, on their characteristics and the parameters of their spaces, not on their individuality, their personality and how they do things on a continuously evolving, everyday basis. Manuals may even be harmful, because they give designers the impression that they have done all they had to do and have considered all there was to consider. But things are definitely not like that. The designer who relies on manuals alone will certainly have omitted the individuality and true reality of life!

Yet manuals are also useful and sometimes indispensable for finding answers about how to proceed after having asked the right questions. Nobody would dream of stopping people in the street to take their measurements. In fact, it would be quite meaningless from a statistical standpoint in any case: luckily for us, we have our manuals!

For many of the answers we need, we do not have to disturb anyone else: we know them ourselves, either because they are the simplest or most common issues, or because we have plenty of case studies in the specific field in question at our disposal.

Other answers call for a tool to help us navigate our way across the endless ocean of information, knowing how to choose and how to rule out the misleading ones (and the web is full of them). The fact is that the challenge on the Internet today is not whether it contains the data we need, but where to find them and how reliable they are.

In addition, complex, specialised issues generally call for input from individuals with specific competence: the knowledge contributed by individuals is always more articulate than the sum total of notions (holism).

3.5   The Five Keys for the Answer

This summary classifies the characteristics of answers under five main headings. Applying these in order will enable you to find the right answer.

1 The right questions deserve an answer

The aim is to construct the answer in a way that responds to the designer's knowledge, his tools and his needs (not an abstract answer, then, but one that is tangibly relevant to the issue at hand and to suitable means and methods). This means that the answer's complexity will vary with the complexity of the issue in question.

2 Can you do that using the "finding the answer" method?

"Finding the right answer" is not an obvious process with no consequences, but a clear, targeted one. To go about "finding the answer", you have to organise your thinking and give it a structure to accelerate things and rule out the wrong answers (which abound in the web). While it is true that there will be no need to search for many of the answers, because they are familiar to the person conducting the search (either because they are the simplest and most common ones, or because there are plenty of precedents to hand), many other answers require a tool to help you find your way around the endless ocean of information. In the case of complex or specialised answers, you may also have to partner with others.

The complexity of the issue may vary considerably and aim at highlighting certain actions (e.g. the difficulty involved in getting up from the toilet), or investigate the adequacy of structures (e.g. grandad coming back home from hospital) or even study how the whole system hangs together (a building, its furniture and its management, e.g. in a specialised structure).

3 The right answer or the best answer?

There is no such thing as the right answer.

There is no such thing as an answer that is good for everybody, because all individuals and all situations are bound to be different. The answers that might be good for everyone (the ones you find in the manuals) would only work if were all tailor's dummies. But since we are not, the answer has to be constructed each time on the basis of the characteristics of the individual, of the place and of the situation.

The solutions available for achieving an objective may be quite different, but all valid: you have to know how to choose.

4 But will I be capable of understanding?

Every individual has his own way of tackling problems, depending on his background and learning, his knowledge and his interests.

The search for answers, especially if they are complex, is an important form of active learning. The same concepts may be found in different areas of knowledge, with different degrees of complexity of approach. The point is to find your own method. Finding the right answer enables you to avoid running up against the block of incomprehensible language when conducting your search: you may find the additional information you need to be accessible and suited to your level of background, learning and interests.

5 Answers come on different levels

To avoid the risk of research getting nowhere, information can be classified according to the level of difficulty involved in understanding it, on a sliding scale of complexity.

Directly applicable answers

These are generally non-specialised answers that are accessible to everyone and formulated in the language of solutions. In other words, they are information that already provides design answers to the question in quantitative or qualitative terms. They generally refer to the simplest of issues (access, reach, required effort etc.) or the application of standards (dimensions, distances, heights etc.). There are certainly manuals and standards that cover this category. The important thing is to understand whether, when and how to apply them. They should always be appraised with a critical eye, however, so as to identify whether, despite complying with standards and regulations, they fail to comply with the concepts of Design for All (respect for human dignity, durability of their characteristics, consistency with management).

Conceptual answers

These are answers that are accessible to those who have acquired a basic level of interdisciplinary understanding (e.g. of the basic terminology of fields other than your own). They often provide data that are not directly related to design and call for a critical appraisal in order for them to be translated into design input and decisions. There may be simplified didactic texts that enable topics to be included in this category that would otherwise be purely specialised (generally speaking, the information provided by associations and intended for patients of a particular pathology are of this kind).

Specialised answers

These are answers that are primarily accessible to those who are familiar with the subject (e.g. it takes a doctor to assess how a given illness may degenerate as time goes by). A designer must have the ability to notice when he needs to acquire specialised information that will be useful for his work (he should not ignore the question as a way of avoiding the difficulty of a complex issue). Yet he must be capable of involving the right specialists in determining clear aims, an art that should never be taken for granted.

Chapter 4
Humanistic Design

The rational approach and the humanistic approach.

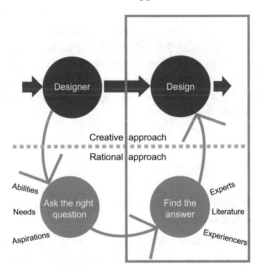

The designer is the last one to act in chain of decision-making, because he is the one who translates the ideas into practical works. Everyone can/must contribute to defining the design decisions, on the basis of the vantage point provided by his or her particular discipline. But in the end it is the designer who defines what will ultimately be made or built. Before this, everyone is entitled to make all the comments and propose all the variables imaginable, but once the designer gets to work, there is no going back.

This is what makes the profession so alluring, but it is also an enormous responsibility.

THINKING ABOUT IT

To clarify the impact that research can have on the final product, I quote the example of what at first sight looks like a rather simple research project: how to determine the right height of a worktop. To reach a conclusion, we have to consider the tasks to be done there, the dimensions of individuals' bodies, the chair, the equipment, how many people will use the worktop, what they will do there and so on. The analysis of each of these parameters will probably lead to a different result from the others. You only have to consider that it

© Springer Nature Switzerland AG 2019
L. Bandini Buti, *Ask the Right Question*,
https://doi.org/10.1007/978-3-319-96346-4_4

might be used by people of very different statures. A good researcher will draw up an interesting document with an analysis of all the variables and will pinpoint all the possible solutions. Research like this is destined to be filed away, because it apparently offers no solutions.

To find the solution, you have to interpret the data and make some decisions. For example, if one of the correct heights of the worktop is determined by the problems encountered by someone sitting in a wheelchair, the data concerning him will take precedence, because he has very little chance to adapt, while someone who is taller can adapt more easily. This means that the right dimension in this case is certainly not an arithmetic average, but the result of a conscious—and often painful—choice. The solution might also lie in other areas concerned with technology (such as adjustable systems) or the organisation of the work-place (by providing different tables and organising the working shifts accordingly).

The answers will often—in fact nearly always—be contradictory. A psychologist will, quite rightly, suggest his own way of seeing things, a technologist another and a doctor yet another. Together, this will create a collage of knowledge to which the designer will respond with his creative decisions. That is where the value lies in multidisciplinary research. It is in this contradictory input that the design process acquires its value of ultimate synthesis that applies creativity to the task of tackling the inevitable contradictions.

4.1   Rational Design

Designing for All does not restrict the designer's creativity; on the contrary, it stimulates it with new challenges.

In order to generate products, places and things for everyone, Design for All instructs us not to look for shortcomings, but for opportunities.

THINKING ABOUT IT

It is very often the shortcomings of a situation that are assessed and considered. We collect observations about what does not function: we complain about the parking spaces reserved for people with disabilities that are occupied by people who are not entitled to use them or about cars that are parked on the pavement. Of course we are right to complain and I understand why those who have to live with the consequences protest. It all encourages people to demonstrate in the street, but it is of little service when it comes to suggesting solutions that might be useful for everyone, even for those who are just tired or lazy or want/have to do something different.

For example, are we really sure that cutlery for people with disabilities does not have the potential to create a different, more convenient way for all of us to handle our food? It would mean eliminating discrimination… and cutting costs.

Designers can/must transform the answers they collect into design input:

- *for the majority of people*

Trying to achieve the greatest possible satisfaction for the largest number of people: that is what you do when you adopt the 50th percentile of anthropometric mea-surements, so as to be certain that you are catering for as many people as possible;

- *opting for a compromise*

Catering for the 50th percentile is not always the right option, however, since you may have to assign a different weight to the abilities of the various categories of individuals, some of whom can adapt better than others.

THINKING ABOUT IT

At what height should light switches be installed in a bedroom? To find a light switch in a dark room, you very often end up stretching your arm out and tapping around on the wall. For this to work, the light switch must be at the expected height, the one that is most often used in bedrooms, regardless of the sophisticated analyses of ergonomics!

The issue of where the light switches should be located, either inside or outside the rooms whose lighting they control, is also highly controversial. If the switches are located inside the rooms, the association between the control and the person controlling is absolutely certain... but you have to tap around in the dark! But if the switch is located outside the room, where it is often associated with other switches, you have to make a choice that may end up being one of trial and error. In addition, you also risk unintentionally switching on the lights in a room without noticing, as often happens to me with the storage closet. The best solution will be the one that the designer considers to be best suited to the specific situation. In a retirement home, for example, he will be more concerned to guarantee certainty of the association between the equipment and the light to be lit, considering the relatively higher frequency of people with cognitive problems.

Why should I raise such an apparently unimportant issue? Because it is a simple example that can help us understand and make us think when we have to tackle more complex situations.

- *choosing the right products*

The range of products available on the market is another factor that has a decisive impact on the accessibility of products and places. By using products that can be adapted to the different conditions required by a variety of situations or tasks, places can be made permanently or temporarily suitable for the different people who will use them or the events that will take place in them.

THINKING ABOUT IT

The Italian word for furniture, *mobile*, is very fitting, since it tells us that the object is intended to be moved around.

Chairs, armchairs and tables are all mobile pieces of furniture that we actually move when we sit down at a table or to relax. Cupboards are also pieces of furniture that get moved around, but not with the same everyday frequency: they usually have to wait until you move house.

The good old drawing board is the ultimate in elasticity: it moves up and down and its inclination can be changed, so it's fine even if you are small and your drawing is big.

- *designing elasticity*

The real challenge when you are designing for all is how to make elasticity into the principle that generates the design in all its aspects of management, technique, plant and décor.

THINKING ABOUT IT

A family is mobile, while a house is immobile. Every change, even the slightest, may be impossible or too costly. It is often our own house that is too rigid, maybe making it moderately suitable for everything, or maybe for nothing at all. An architect who designs houses before knowing who is going to live in them can do nothing but envisage them for generic users. It will then be up to the inhabitants to adapt themselves to it.[1]

So why don't we design an 'elastic house' that would adapt to our everyday needs, to our exceptional requests (such as organising a party, all of us together) and even to our needs for more drastic adaptations, such as making the bathroom a little bigger so that there's room for grandad to use his wheelchair?

We should never be afraid of what seems to be obvious. In actual fact, what appears to be obvious often conceals what we think we know but in reality do not.

4.2   Humanistic Design

Creativity is the tool wielded by the designer

Many authors, especially those with an Anglo-Saxon mindset, give the impression that, once you have received your answers, the design has found its sense of direction and can forge ahead with certainty. It's almost as though you could just feed the data into a computer that would process them and come up with the best solution.

This is the rational/pragmatic approach to design.

My approach, on the other hand, is that once you have your answers, the next necessary step is an important phase of appraisal that takes absolutely nothing for granted. That's because, as I already mentioned, the answers are certainly bound to be contradictory. Nor could it be otherwise in a multidisciplinary process, where every individual contributes his or her knowledge and diversified skills. And what I say is not restricted to the specialists alone, but also takes in all sorts of others: those who will use the product of the design process, but also those who will manage it, maintain it, dismantle it or profit from it.

---

[1]The architect Giancarlo De Carlo was the first in Italy (in 1970) to design participatory public housing together with the future residents in the Matteotti neighbourhood of Terni, encountering considerable difficulties with the bureaucrats who were disoriented by the revolutionary new concept.

This is the humanistic/creative approach to design.

THINKING ABOUT IT

Knowing how to do things, knowing how to have things done, knowledge.

Designing 'for All' must involve all the disciplines necessary for understanding the instrumental, human and behavioural aspects of the interaction between man and products in the physical and social environment. This calls for the people involved to be capable of managing a multidisciplinary design process. Participation is the tool that makes a dialogue possible between the various disciplines and skills necessary for a correct, conscious design.

In order to operate in a multidisciplinary group, every member of the group must:

- know how to do the things that are part of his own specialisation. In other words, the expert must be competent and attentive in his profession as an architect, a technician, a health worker, an entrepreneur, a civil servant, an administrator and so on and must keep himself constantly up to date;
- know how to have things done; in other words, know how to channel and organise what others are capable of doing better (because it is their job), co-ordinating them synergically to achieve their objectives;
- know; in other words, be in possession of the tools, the vocabulary and the basic notions of the other disciplines involved, so as to be able to dialogue with others consciously. And also to be able to tackle those decision-making and productive structures that tend to hide behind the inevitable shield of saying "it cannot be done", the shield that is always held up against innovation by structures and people who fear change![2]

The solutions available for achieving the aim of the design process may be quite varied, yet all valid; the designer's task is to find the best conscious choice, which means a constructive compromise.

Speaking of compromise, my colleagues are sometimes scandalised by the concept, because the word is often perceived with a negative inference, although it does express the fact quite well that this conscious choice is never entirely painless.

Every time you make a choice, you discard others.

THINKING ABOUT IT

Engineers look for the right object, because they know that only one is right. That's what they are taught at university. And it is true, because if you want to achieve a given effect, there is certainly one solution that is better than others in terms of cost, reliability, performance and so on.

Architects and designers deal in compromises, on the other hand, because there is always an endless range of solutions for dealing with every issue. That's partly because some of those issues refuse to be merely rational. There are no objective parameters for measuring such things as the quality of aesthetics and of form or the perception of reliability, for example. The only way to assess them is through our feelings. That's why I call this 'humanistic' design, as opposed to pragmatic, rational design.

Another way of looking at this is to remember that human beings appreciate more than mere utility, otherwise there would be no way of explaining why, when our prehistoric ancestors made pottery recipients for transporting liquids, they covered them with 'useless' geometric patterns.

---

[2] C. P.Odescalchi, L. Bandini Buti, G. Cortili, E. Moretti *La concezione ergonomica, le condizioni di attuazione, il suo contributo alla prevenzione*, ECSC document N° 1654/75.

Engineers give objects their utility, while designers give poetry to utility and artists give us poetry.

I already mentioned that designers are asked to design for the future. Nobody wants a car that is designed to suit today's taste but that will age and date quickly. To make things more difficult, change has accelerated even more just lately: just think of how much our personal relationships have changed in the last twenty years with the spread of the mobile telephone, or what will happen when self-driving cars become the norm.

THINKING ABOUT IT

In the automobile industry, every manufacturer focuses his research these days on self-driving cars.

But the question for us is how can designers hypothesise the kind of behaviour, needs and expectations that we shall have in relation to something that is not yet part of our lives? The classical tools of research can tell us precious little and what they can tell us is unreliable. If we ask the man in the street, his answers will be dictated by hopes and fears that are also of negligible use.

Designers will have to project their thinking into the future and ask themselves questions, the right questions. How will people spend their time in the car when it drives itself? Will it be comparable to how we spend our time now in a train or a plane, or shall we still want to keep an eye on our route? Will there be intelligent cars devoted to tourism, for example, that will take us to visit the places that interest us? Or shall we simply drive our cars as in the past and then just ask them to find themselves a parking space and tell us where they are? Or will it only be easy to use the automatic facility when we are on a motorway? Designers can only answer all these questions if they are familiar with design discipline, of course, but also only if they have learned to observe the world. In a nutshell, if they have developed a cultural foundation to their work.

That's what I always tell my students.

Part II
How It Functions

Chapter 5
The Evolution of Accessible Design

5.1 The Evolution of the Machine

In complex products, regardless of the scale of their production (small runs or large series), ergonomic design research sets out to cater for the new demands of inter-disciplinarity of approach and in particular seems to have become indispensable for developing high-risk objects with a high degree of technological content, i.e. those objects that call for such massive investments that the risk of failure must be reduced to a minimum, or those objects in which the system is so critical that even the slightest lack of correspondence between man and machine may cause damage out of all proportion to the scale of the anomalous event that produced it. Malfunctions are notoriously often caused by 'misunderstandings' between a technological system and the humans who govern it. Many of the accidents that are attributed to 'human error' are actually brought about by such 'misunderstandings' that occur when people react instinctively to an unexpected event or a particularly stressful situation in ways that deviate from the models they have learned. Many accidents, even the most disastrous ones, can be traced back to such misunderstandings between man and machine, to inadequate legibility or comprehensibility of signals and messages or to the difficulty involved in learning or remembering the correct procedures to be followed.

THINKING ABOUT IT

A famous aircraft accident happened years ago during landing because the pilots had switched off the engine that was functioning correctly and left on the one that had a fault. The one with the fault had burst into flame during take-off and had been switched off promptly. The pilots saw smoke coming into their cabin from the starboard side and were certain that the starboard engine was the one with the fault. They were so sure that they relied on their perception, even though the displays told them otherwise. In actual fact, the smoke was being relayed by a draught. When the time came to land, they opened the

© Springer Nature Switzerland AG 2019
L. Bandini Buti, *Ask the Right Question*,
https://doi.org/10.1007/978-3-319-96346-4_5

throttle on the port engine, but nothing happened: it was the one that was in flames! It's worth noting that all the passengers and the in-flight personnel knew which engine had the fault... they could see it giving off smoke, but nobody asked them. The pilots had relied on their natural perception, which tends to take over at times of great stress.

One particularly useful, albeit extreme, case is that of space travel, when the only way that the efficiency of products and systems can be checked directly is under the notably artificial conditions of simulation. If the input of the humanities were to be made only when the technological design has been defined, the scope for introducing it in the overall design would be very limited—and that would be extremely risky in such a critical sector. This explains why human input has always been introduced throughout the design process, in a continuous exchange between hypotheses and checks. Much of the ergonomics that we know today was actually developed in fields of this kind, where it has played a major role.

The dialogue between individuals and systems has evolved with the passage of time, progressing from a natural process to an ever-increasing degree of codification.

Natural information

If we analyse how machines develop, paying special attention to how the system of relations and information with the human being who manages the machines evolves, we can see that simple machines express their functions mostly through sensory channels, with no mediation.

When the blacksmith sees the red-hot iron he is working on, its colour gives him all the information he needs about how malleable it is and how much energy he needs to apply to forge it. The farm worker feels the need to sharpen his sickle when it starts to grow less efficient. The presence and quantity of active energy is self-evident when the motor is man himself, as it is when the potter turns his wheel, and it is still evident when the motion is transmitted by the cogs in a mill or by a motor powered by drive belts. Even today, the noise generated by a system that is running provides a great deal of information about how it is functioning, so much so that our hearing is still irreplaceable for certain processes of fine-tuning, such as in sports cars.

Simple codified information

At a later stage, as machines' performances increased and with the advent of technology, the need arose to add useful information in all those cases where basic sensory perception could not be used. This is what happened for example when the need arose to know the pressure of a liquid inside a tank, the load that could be borne by a conduit, the intensity of the current absorbed by a motor or the temperature of a liquid, all things that cannot be perceived with the senses and must be read off an instrument that transforms the information into values measured on appropriate scales, so translates the condition we want to know about into codified information. We also have to remember that natural information can often be too approximate to be of any operational use. Experience tells us that water has reached 100 °C when it boils and that tells us that it is time to add the pasta. But this kind of sensory information is often insufficient, because we also need to know other intermediate values of the temperature or how the process is proceeding and when a certain event can be expected to happen. So we need to know and use codes that are more specific than our sensory perception.

In the kitchen, we can observe the difference between an ordinary saucepan and a pressure cooker. With the ordinary pan, we can use our senses to judge how the cycle is proceeding, how far the food has been cooked and whether we need to do anything or add anything: I can hear the water boiling and can add ingredients, stir the contents and use my sight, my sense of smell and my taste to keep check. The process falls within the scope of common natural perceptions. With the pressure cooker, I have to rely exclusively on codified information or on my own experience, which is also expressed in a codified manner. I may say that "the food will be ready to eat in 32 minutes", but I shall only know afterwards if the information was correct. The difference is substantial, because I use my senses in the first case, but in the second I use abstract codes.

THINKING ABOUT IT

When measuring instruments were first introduced, the model of the man-machine relationship was still basically the natural one, with just a few additions. The information system had not really come about at that stage, except in aircraft. For this reason, as instruments were considered an appendage of our basic natural perception, they tended to be located on the spot where the phenomenon took place: the voltmeter and the ammeter were close to the motor, the pressure gauge on the tank, the thermometer on the basin. Until not so long ago the coolant water thermometer used to be located on the radiator cap in many cars. When that is how things are organised, the operator has to know the cycle and the technology to be able to operate on the basis both of non-mediated sensory information and of codified information.

Complex codified information

As systems become more complex to govern, remote controls are introduced, operations are mechanised and, lastly, computerisation takes hold, they all contribute to move the operator gradually away from the process, which he is no longer expected to operate directly, because he is now specialised in managing the system. This has made work increasingly abstract and purely technical information redundant, since the engineer, as pragmatic as ever, has channelled all the machinery's phenomena onto his screen, so that the screen is now the representation of the technological system and no importance is attributed to representing the system that the operator has in mind. Control panels fill up with pressure, temperature and speed readings and run the risk of becoming not more usable, but more abstract.

It was at this stage that ergonomics developed its contribution for progressing from the purely technological representation of the process to the definition of the information necessary, sufficient and comprehensible to the operator at various moments, by analysing the technological cycle, man's characteristics and limitations, his training and the information at his disposal, so as to be in a position to design information and control systems corresponding to them.

THINKING ABOUT IT

Had you noticed (did you know?) that the screens on aircraft flight decks are mostly analogical? This configuration enables the normal condition of the various screens to be arranged vertically, so that any anomalies stand out instantly at a glance. Just imagine how difficult it would be to get an overall impression if the system only gave a series of mutually incomprehensible numerical readings!

The designer's responsibilities are also changing radically, for now mostly in areas concerned primarily with automating the production processes and computerising the design processes, but they will soon also extend to a much broader field of activities. Designers will be expected above all to command a capacity for creative synthesis of complex technological issues, which will call for new capacities and knowledge that has expanded to encompass specific methods and less extemporary approaches to creativity.

THINKING ABOUT IT

One question still remains unanswered for now: is it possible to conceive of a design process using nothing but IT media, i.e. by sketching on a computer? This is what today's students tend to do: forgetting how to use the pencil, they are enthusiastic, galvanised and indeed made a little lazy by computers. What I tell them is that it is indispensable to use the pencil, not as a way of remembering the good old days or out of nostalgia, but as a real need, since it is only when you sketch with a pencil that you have the necessary degree of indeterminacy of your thinking as it takes shape. A computer expects you to provide it with such things as the radius of a curve, the nature of a surface, the dimensions of the object and a degree of precision immediately, well before they actually become significant issues, diverting your attention away from your specific focus on creativity. This is certainly how things stand today... but tomorrow? Maybe there will be tools capable of operating following the degree of indeterminacy of human thinking as it takes shape.

5.2   The Phases of the Design Project

The phases and activities necessary for developing a product, from the intangible idea to the final prototype and then on to serial production, are likely to vary with the nature of the object in question, of the size of the series to be produced, of the level of technology and automation in the production process, of the size of the target market, of the scale and diversification of the target population and of its degree of education and familiarity with the use of the category into which the object falls.

Some passages are always typical and indispensable, however: the intangible phase, the model phase and the prototype phase.

The intangible phase

In a first phase, the object we want to develop takes the shape of an intangible idea, because it comprises writings, images and graphic and/or virtual representations. At this stage there are very few possibilities of putting the idea to the test of real people for the purpose of getting feedback from them about how they might use an object that does not yet exist. D. A. Norman says that it is unlikely that individuals will be capable of evaluating innovation, because they would have to imagine something of which they have no experience.

The model phase

This is the phase when the idea can already be represented by 3D models (of the whole or its parts), whose main characteristic is their ability to represent its dimensions well, although they can say little or nothing about its finishes or how it will function. While such non-functioning models enable us to conduct certain user tests with individuals, they do not enable us to offer a complete experience of using the object (for example the actions of getting into and out of a car that call for a complete model, or the qualities of a grip that depend on how the surfaces are finished and the degree of grip[1] of the materials used, or again the quality of noise generated or of efforts required, which can only be evaluated when an object has been finished and mounted on the structures where it will have its ultimate home). This means that the sample of individuals interviewed cannot be made up of ordinary people, but must be selected in such a way as to stimulate a mental picture of real conditions of use, i.e. people who are capable of mental abstraction.

> THINKING ABOUT IT
>
> A model, which is often made with cheap materials, such as cardboard, is also indispensable for starting to get a tangible idea of the object's real dimensions. When I started out on my career (I was still a student), I had the chance to design an ordinary tomb and, like any good enthusiastic beginner, I filled it with all sorts of beautiful details.
>
> A disaster.
>
> Some poor chiseller had to struggle to create little holes with a drill where I had imagined the sense of transparency of the passage between life and death… Luckily, I was young, but I learned a lesson that I was never to forget.

The prototype phase

The third phase is the one when prototypes can be made that function or can be used for making analyses with real individuals in conditions of real use. Experience teaches us that even when we use functioning prototypes it may not be very easy to run tests with an ordinary cross-section of people, either because the manufacturer wants to keep the secret of a product that has not yet been launched on the market, or for reasons of safety with products that have not yet been approved by the standards authorities.

---

[1]By grip we mean the resistance that a surface offers to a moving hand. A typical example is a tailor-made rubber surface with a minimal angle of a sloping surface that enables the sample to slide.

Finished products

When we start having the first finished products available, they can be tested by ordinary individuals during their everyday activities. Here we have the highest quality of subjective response, but no possibility to modify the product any more. This practice has often developed, despite having no immediate advantages, because it furnishes important input for creating the next generation of new products.

Summary

These observations can be summarised in a diagram, whose purpose is to establish when and how real individuals can be used to obtain their appraisals, but at times when their observations can still have a real influence on the product's development.

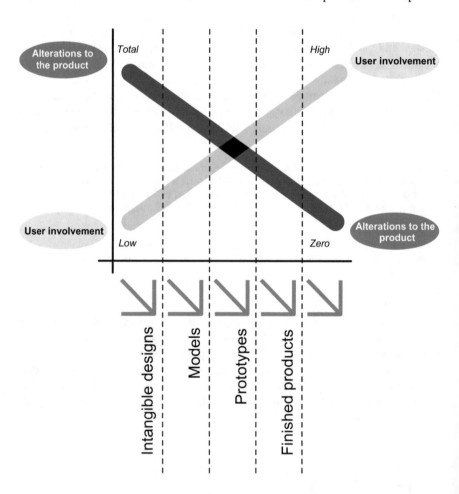

On the horizontal axis, the diagram has the various phases of the design's development, from the intangible idea to serial production, while on its vertical axis is the possibility to modify the product and involve users. At the beginning of the process, the possibility to modify the product is highest, because no definitive decisions have yet been made, while at the end of the process only very marginal alterations will be allowed. Vice versa, it is very difficult to obtain any reactions in the first phases from users who have no tangible products to experience, something that only becomes possible when the product is finished and functioning.

It should be remembered that if a correct ergonomic design process is not embarked on from the very start of the design activity, i.e. if you wait until you have prototypes available before you start running any tests with individuals, the possibility of making a difference to the product's design is very limited, if not irrelevant. This means that subjective investigations call for the use of specific techniques that change with the development phase reached by the design process.

THINKING ABOUT IT

Everybody at Fiat agreed that the subjective reaction of the individual who was to buy and use the car was a vital issue to bear in mind. But since they were all good engineers, they insisted that it had to be done seriously, i.e. when the first prototypes were available. When I asked whether it would be possible to make the car 3 cm higher, they told me not to say daft things. That is why I built this diagram to be on the same wavelength as the engineers: its effect was to introduce forms of user analysis into the design project other than those restricted to real people testing the car on the road.

5.3 Man's Artefacts

The Evolution of the Car

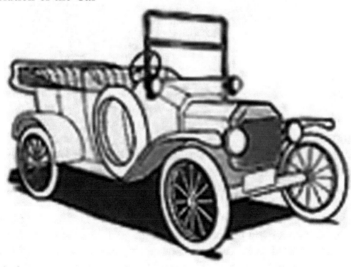

First period

It Moves

Model T Ford—1908

Complex products like cars, aircraft, trains or many means of production, have experienced a process of developing from simple objects to highly sophisticated objects.

One excellent example of this is the development of the motor car.

***

In the early days, all that was expected was that the car would move without the aid of horses. It also took you to your destination with a reasonable degree of safety.

And it retained many signs of the now-redundant horse, such as its drive power, which is still expressed today in horsepower. And we still also talk of the car's coachwork.

Instead of a coachman, who also used to have to take care of the animals, we now had a chauffeur, who had to take care of the workings of the mechanical beast.

Like the coachman, the chauffeur sat out in front, exposed to the elements, while those who rode behind had the benefit of a protective hood, just as in a coach… after all, they were the bosses!

The automobile (auto … mobile, i.e. capable of moving on its own) moved without horses and was a miracle!

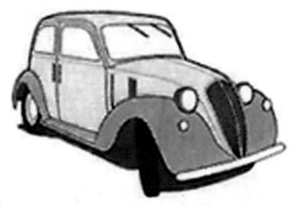

Second period

It Protects You

Fiat 1100 (108C) 1938

The time duly arrived when it was taken for granted that the car moved on its own (without horses) and that anyone could drive it. But not women… that would still have been a step too far… the driver had to be a man and also quite a strong one.

By now there was no distinction between the driver and the driven any more: everyone, both driver and passengers, had to be protected from the elements. The vehicle was expected to be capable of protecting them from atmospheric agents, from the wind, from freezing conditions and from the direct sun. This led to the classical saloon car, with certain characteristics that seem prehistorical these days. Somebody noticed, for example, that there was a free source of heat under the bonnet and attempts were made—successfully—to make use of it in cold weather.

THINKING ABOUT IT
My first 1100 had no heating, so in the winter I had to kit myself out with an overcoat, gloves and a scarf. My aunts asked me "Why do you use the car when it's so cold? Wait for spring!"

In these cars, changing gear was hard work because synchromesh gear changes had not yet been invented. The system was based on a pair of satellites that moved to the right and left and forwards and backwards (some of you will remember how the gears would crash!). Hence the 'H' shaped layout that mechanical gear changes still have today, a purely technological and now prehistorical configuration. But if the gear lever was hard, what could be done to make it softer? It was made longer, using one of the first laws of physics. But to be effective, the gear lever had to be so long that it reached half way to the passenger seat when the car was put into reverse… which was a good excuse for gallantly lengthening a hand towards a girl seated next to you (as much as we were allowed in those dark days).

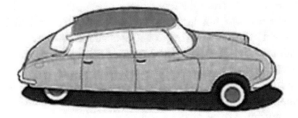

Third period

Comfort

Citroën DS 1955

At the end of the Second World War, in the midst of the return to a quality lifestyle, Citroën revolutionised the car by creating a truly 'auto-mobile drawing room' with every accessory for a comfortable, silent journey: ultra-comfortable seats and hydro-pneumatic suspension with a variable height and resistance.

In those days, it was not unusual to pass a car parked by the roadside, while carsick children vomited, because the way the vehicle bounced was very similar to the stomach's own rhythm and easily caused freshly-eaten food to be regurgitated. In those days, the Renault ergonomics centre was busy studying the interaction between the elasticity of the tyres, of the suspension and of the seating, in order to find a solution to this problem.

THINKING ABOUT IT

I had one of these cars and it was a game for my children to help me open the doors. When the car's engine was off, the car settled right down so that the door would knock against the kerbstone. The game was to send the children to the other side and have them lean out like a sidecar to make the car slope in that direction and free the door. They really enjoyed it!

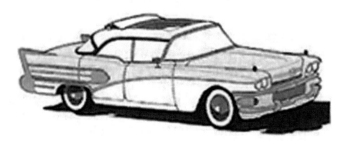

Fourth period

It Surprises You

A typical American car from the late fifties

By now, the car was not just a means of transport, but had become a status symbol. In the USA in the fifties, cars changed look every year, exactly like clothing fashions. It was the American dream. And you might come in for criticism if you were still driving a 1955 Buick in 1956.

These cars were living rooms with extremely powerful, low-performance and high-consumption engines, applying the principle that 'if petrol is cheap, all you have to do is consume a lot of it'.

The front seat was a three-seater bench, so offered no protection against slipping sideways. But the gear lever was right in the middle of the living room space. To keep that space clear, the dashboard lever was invented, although it was a real insult to normal mechanical logic.

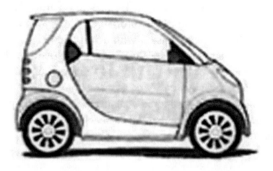

Fifth period

It Is Like You

SMART 1996

Lastly, and most recently, cars have been designed to cater for the needs of specific niches of users—and not only in terms of performance. A good example of this is the SMART, which created an image and a lifestyle. One typical characteristic of this car—and one that was new to the auto scene—is that it is two-tone. That does not mean that it is painted in a variety of colours like cars were in the USA in the fifties, but that its structure has been in two colours from the very start. These days, single-tone SMARTs are practically only for courtesy cars or for shy people.

And what might the future hold? Maybe self-driving cars? One obstacle that will not be easy to overcome will be who pays if there is an accident, which at the moment seems to be an almost insuperable objection.

I am convinced that the first self-driving cars will be ordinary cars with drivers, who will ask the car to find itself a parking space once they have arrived at their destination, and then to keep them informed. Another possible option is that the car will be an ordinary city car, but once it reaches the motorway it will go where you tell it, maybe at a speed dictated by our often absurd road signs … but at least you will be able to sleep in peace.

Chapter 6
Ergonomics in Italy

First class workers and second class workers

All over Europe (and also in other places) in the seventies, dangerous work was entrusted to foreign migrant workers (Gastarbeiter) who tended not to be members of trade unions. These 'second class' workers would spend a few years working in a factory and then go back home. Since Italy had not yet experienced foreign immigration, but only a massive shift of working population from the south to the north of the country, we only had 'first class' workers. For this reason, the solution to environmental problems in Italy was not the turnover of migrant workers, but the need to design healthy environments.

THINKING ABOUT IT

In those years, I was invited to express an opinion in a factory making car batteries in the south of France. The workers, who were all Algerians, handled the lead directly, running the known risk of contracting saturnism.[1] However, the workers spent several years living in prefabricated housing near the factory and generally did not stay long enough to contract the disease in serious form.

But then France enacted a new law that obliged firms to employ at least 10% of its workforce from French citizens. But nobody wanted to work under those conditions. The whole approach to production had to be turned on its head to cater for the 'first class' workers.

But let's get back to Italian ergonomics: it is not commonly known that Italian ergonomics has played an important role on the international scene.

Ergonomics was only introduced to Italy in 1970, a good 20 years after it was first formulated elsewhere. It started by tackling high-risk workplaces, as in other European countries, but without the support of any university structures, unlike France or the UK.

Things did not look so promising at the outset.

Things changed in 1970, when the Italian Parliament passed a law known as the Workers' Statute, which guaranteed workers' rights in the areas of trade union

---

[1]Saturnism is chronic poisoning caused by lead and its compounds: it is a professional illness whose symptoms are anaemia, stomach pains, pains in the joints, paralysis and sometimes also nervous disturbances and epileptic fits.

© Springer Nature Switzerland AG 2019
L. Bandini Buti, *Ask the Right Question*,
https://doi.org/10.1007/978-3-319-96346-4_6

membership, social security and health and provided for the establishment of representative worker councils in factories. But above all it paved the way for the law to control the conditions of workplaces, also by employing experts.[2] Before this law was passed, the standard practice was to 'monetise the risk', making payments called 'risk indemnities' to workers affected by dangerous working environments. After the law had been passed, the trade unions proposed a plan that was to mark a sea-change in workplace management, encapsulated effectively in the slogan coined in those days: "*la salute non si paga*" (health is not for sale). Employers were pushed by trade union demands to take steps to change the working environment and the workplace, tackling the need to improve and modify working conditions by conducting fact-finding investigations about the potential harmfulness for human health of the environment and the activities taking place in them.

6.1   The Seventies and Eighties: The Industrial Workplace

While there was talk of ergonomics in Italy throughout the sixties, it came across as something of a luxury for rich countries. Those were the years when Italy's post-war economic boom was drawing to a close, a period when the country had focused entirely on development and on its effort to produce... without bothering much about the human cost. So when ergonomics was applied, it was primarily on an individual basis, in the form of studies, contacts and theoretical research, almost entirely in the fields of anthropometrics, of the physiology of labour, of industrial hygiene and of labour medicine. Nevertheless, these theoretical investigations already bore the seed of objectives that would induce this discipline to involve a broader number of others.

The end of the sixties brought the first experiences in factories that were inspired by the need to draw up analytical methods for identifying conditions of risk and consequently developing projects for change. One reason why this happened was the difficulty encountered in reconciling the approach adopted by corporate

---

[2]The law commonly known as the Workers' Statute went onto the Italian statue book on 20 May 1970, was identified with the number 300 for that years and bears the long title of "A law governing the freedom and the dignity of workers, the freedom of trade unions and of trade union activity in the workplace and placement". Article 9 provides that "workers (...) are entitled to control the application of the law for preventing accidents and professional illnesses and to promote the research, elaboration and actuation of all measures suitable for safeguarding their health and their physical integrity".

From the very beginning, ergonomics has generated intense cultural debate. In the course of time, this has enabled certain philosophical principles to take hold that now furnish its conceptual skeleton. These principles state that ergonomics is a discipline that aims at change (i.e. at the design project) and is thus closely related to the process of actuation, and that its application is influenced by stimuli coming from the real outside world: while at one time, the design assumption was that "the factory breeds death", it gradually evolved into "the factory breeds illness", then "work breeds alienation" and ultimately "there is more to life than just organised work".

management and technicians with that of their workers, since industrial relations were fraught with strife in those years. The object of the research comprised a field that had hitherto been tackled only in part or sometimes completely neglected by the study of labour medicine: the postures adopted by workers in relation to the machinery they operated and the production tools they used, the appraisal of the cost in terms of the energy required for each individual operation, the appraisal of the parameters for quantifying heat stress and the distribution of information throughout a given space and for a given time. However it also included an attempt to draw up a methodology for acquiring comprehensive knowledge about the conditions of production that tended to cause 'chronic fatigue'. This phase was marked by the realisation of the importance, for ergonomic purposes, of the analysis of situations at work, although the impact of the trade unions' cultural work and struggle approach on the appraisal of conditions of risk meant that issues of participation and of subjective evaluation tended to play a greater role than structural issues.

This explains why there was a greater focus on environmental issues in Italy compared to the rest of Europe and the degree of primacy they enjoyed. In addition, this was also the period when Italy started feeling the powerful impact of technological modernisation, which brought substantial investments in major plant and depended on the ability to work constantly and at full capacity, without production rates being restricted by external factors that were hard to control, such as issues related to the working environment, its rhythms, mistakes and wastage.

While most attention was focused on high-risk workplaces (such as steelworks and mines) at the beginning of the seventies, these were followed in due course by industrial workplaces, as a consequence of environmental issues (noise, pollution, posture...). Because of these factors, ergonomics started enjoying a degree or prestige in those years as an approach with the characteristics for analysing the reciprocal relationships between man and the environment and for designing the changes necessary as a consequence.

These conditions laid the groundwork for extensive, detailed experimentation in the field of ergonomic methodology for designing machinery, the workplace and the working environment.

As increasing attention came to be paid to the quality of life on the international scene, the seventies brought conditions favourable to the introduction of ergonomics in the working world to Italy. An important push came from the research projects and funding backed by the Social Affairs Division of the European Coal and Steel Community, which aimed to improve working conditions in the steelmaking and mining industries.

Ergonomics now started tackling the industrial working environment in more general terms. This was the period, for example, when several design projects were conducted in the working environment and the workplace in the printing industry.

In this industry, the huge typographic machines used to print newspapers and the rotogravure machines used to print magazines were beset by a host of problems, especially with regard to the issues of noise and of the pollution caused by solvents and by paper dust. The manufacturers of printing machines, where Italian industry played a major role, were concerned to maintain a continuous process of improvement of their products' technical performance, targeting ever-faster printing speeds, so as to increase the number of copies turned out per hour. But these targets could hardly ever be achieved in practice, because the levels of noise and of pollution in the printing works were so high that agreements had to be reached with the trade unions to reduce the printing speed, since that was the only way that the quality of the working environment could be improved in those days. So although the machinery was theoretically capable of functioning perfectly at full capacity, the combination between man and machine did not allow it. This set the stage for the entry of applied ergonomics, which dealt with optimising the relationship between man and the machine and used interdisciplinary analyses and pilot experiments to enable radical improvements to be made that solved many of the problems faced by the printing industry.

Our group was given the task of tackling this problem. One of the most serious environmental issues to be solved was the presence in the air of toluene, the solvent used in printer's inks. Each of the printing machines in the production units bore a notice that specified the maximum speed that could be reached by that specific machine if it was to comply with the company's employment contract agreed with the trade unions. These values had been calculated experimentally, with the aim of keeping the pollution rates within tolerable limits. In many cases, the speed specified for the machine was half that of full capacity, meaning that two machines rather than one had to be employed to achieve a full print run. When you are working to print a weekly magazine, there is clearly no option to lengthen the printing times or postpone the complete run to a later date: either the magazine comes out on time, or it doesn't come out at all.

The problem was tackled starting from the principle that toluene is a very heavy gas that tends to settle near the ground. And yet the many ventilators that had been installed at ground level had had no effect. Why was this? Everyone knew that toluene is very heavy and that it settles at the bottom of a test tube... in the laboratory. Yet despite this knowledge of physics and chemistry, nobody had been able to come up with the answers necessary to solve the printing industry's environmental problem. What was missing? Certainly not funds or laboratories, of which there was no shortage in the firms that manufactured these highly specialised machines. And certainly not the economic return on investment, because the demand for acceptable working conditions was making this activity socially burdensome and economically unsustainable. Everyone wanted a solution, but nobody could find one.

The mistake that had been made was to believe that the best place for analyses and experiments was the laboratory: with its perfect, controlled conditions and certain, constant monitoring, it was the paradise of the researchers and academics who like to have data with two zeros after the decimal point.

Luckily for us from the Society for Applied Ergonomics, we tended to have a heavy hands-on approach (which is why we were looked upon with suspicion!).

THINKING ABOUT IT

It should come as a surprise to nobody that the problem of the working environment in the rotogravure printing industry had not yet been solved, despite major investments and the force of very active corporate research in the laboratories in Italy, the country that led the field in this printing technology. In fact, when we went to visit Cerutti in Casale Monferrato[3] to ask for technological support to help us solve certain structural issues, we were told that no country in the world considered the problems we were discussing and, since the company produced mostly for export, it was not interested in following us along that particular path. We were told that we should not go away thinking that other countries had no noise or toluene, but they did not constitute a problem there, because the workers employed in the areas at greatest risk in Germany came from Turkey, in France they came from Algeria, in the UK they came from India, Pakistan and other countries, in the USA they were Latinos and blacks. Only in Italy did we have no throwaway second class workers, with the result that we had these problems and they remained unsolved.

These were the reasons that obliged us as Italian ergonomists to set to work designing healthy environments, unlike what happened in other European countries.[4]

Solving the enigma of the toluene that did not settle on the ground was not easy, but in the end we understood what was happening.

The printing machines were enormous beasts, more than five metres tall and stretching at least 25 metres in length. At the foot, they were fitted with powerful suction grills, designed by German technicians from MAN,[5] which were based on the principle that toluene, being heavy, should settle on the ground, so that is where it should be collected and eliminated.

But the fact was that toluene did not behave in the working environment in the same way as in the laboratory: it did not settle on the ground, or actually it did try to settle there, but the production process had the effect of heating the air (which made it tend to rise), while the paper was whizzing upwards at speeds of nearly 100 km/h, dragging the air up with it.

Once we had unravelled the enigma, all we had to do as a first step was switch the suction system off to achieve a substantial reduction in the level of environmental pollution. The expensive suction system was actually harmful.

And that is where the difference lies between theory and operational practice.

As a result of this, Italian ergonomics started enjoying considerable prestige in that period as an approach that had the characteristics necessary for analysing the reciprocal relationships between man and the environment and for designing the changes made necessary as a consequence.

---

[3]Officine Meccaniche Giovanni Cerutti S.p.A. is an Italian public company based in Casale Monferrato, in the province of Alessandria, that works in the area of designing and building printing machinery and equipment, mostly for rotogravure and flexography.

[4]For the originality of its contribution to research about the working environment, the Society for Applied Ergonomics won the ADI Compasso d'Oro in 1981 for its research project entitled "Ergonomic Design—Research Applied to Rotogravure Printing Machines" (workplace, working environment, atmospheric pollution, energy consumption, levels of productivity), group leader L. Bandini Buti with G. Cortili, F. De Nigris, E. Moretti.

[5]Manroland AG is a German manufacturer based in Augsburg, Offenbach am Main and Plauen, producing printing systems for newspapers and magazines.

This was why the Director of the Conservatoire National des Arts et Métiers in Paris, where ergonomics has been taught for years, sent us one of his assistants, these days we would say an intern, to understand how it was that we managed to design and achieve the improvement of the working environment, while they, academic colossus that they were, produced nothing but concepts. The difference was that we were a really interdisciplinary group of designers, physicists, chemists and doctors and not only theorists

6.2   The Eighties and Nineties: The Tertiary Sector and Services

By the time the nineties came around, improved living conditions and health, longer life expectancy and above all the demand for better living standards combined to ensure that the kinds of interests that had by then been consolidated were now joined by the demand for quality of products and services. An increasingly clear perception was taking hold that the concept of work could and should also encompass all human activities, including the ones related to leisure pursuits, housework and the habitat in general.

While in the early days, in the seventies, attention had been focused primarily on high-risk working environments (steelworks and mines), followed by industrial workplaces for their environmental issues (noise, pollution, posture…), the eighties saw attention shifting to a focus on the tertiary sector and office work, as the IT revolution started to take hold.

In industrial concerns, the steps taken in the seventies had brought tangible improvements to working environments, but above all they had provided operative tools and created a culture of remedial intervention that also started being applied successfully by firms' technical organisms. The more harmful processes were either eliminated because they were economically unsustainable (like the chrome-plating processes that were still a ubiquitous feature of car manufacturing in the sixties) or completely automated, so that human beings were effectively moved away from the sources of pollution. Drastic reductions also started to be made to physical effort, as widespread use was made of lifting and handling mechanisms. The result of all this was a fall in demand for ergonomic research in the industrial sector.

At the same time, the reduction in numbers of people working in manufacturing industry was counterbalanced by an enormous upsurge in those working in the tertiary sector: office work in particular was changing at a very fast pace, driven by the spread of new technologies.[6] The computerised office was here to stay, as was the robotised factory. Since important investments started being made in the

---

[6]The march of the forty thousand Fiat middle management and clerical workers was a demonstration that took place in Turin on 14 October 1980. Thousands of middle management and clerical staff working for the auto manufacturer Fiat took to the streets of central Turin to protest against the belief that office work should be considered a cushy job of privileges, seated in

technology necessary for these computerised offices, they required to be used for work at maximum capacity, just as had happened to manufacturing industry a few decades earlier: nobody could afford to allow humanity to be the limiting factor.

The ergonomic approach was now called on less and less to intervene in situations of physical effort or pollution, but increasingly in conditions of mental fatigue, stress and the quality of information. As more and more people were working in the tertiary sector, the evidence mounted that it was a false presumption that these activities did not generate any difficulties for human being because they took place in places that were clean, well-lit and with low noise levels, and that the classical problems afflicting the working environment did not apply here, because office work constituted a condition of social privilege. On the contrary: the realisation dawned that working in the tertiary sector can be harmful because it obliges people to adopt a fixed posture, puts much stress on their eyesight and above all is mentally demanding.

6.3   The Nineties: Design

Practically all of the cases in which ergonomics was involved in Italy in its first twenty years were focused on correcting and improving previous situations where damage had already been done and where it was possible to apply methodologies based on field analyses. What emerged with clarity during that phase was that interventions of correction after the event are difficult and expensive and above all that the damage has already been done.

This led to the realisation that real prevention is generated when the intervention takes place during the design process, before the harmful event has had a chance to happen, by developing appropriate methodologies of forecasting. As a result, ergonomics was involved in this period—first sporadically, then with increasing regularity—not only in the process of analysis, but also in that of designing buildings, machines, products and IT systems.

It was in this phase that ergonomics offered its services as a discipline well-suited to appraising the relationship between the object being designed and the human being destined to use it, generating interest among manufacturers and designers, who started using it primarily for the assistance it could offer in the field of anthropometrics, ultimately subscribing to the equation *Ergonomics = Anthropometrics*, which is actually a narrow view of the discipline.

These days, ergonomics is becoming involved increasingly in all the phases that contribute to defining a design project.

Because it is essentially methodological, the ergonomic approach lends itself to being applied to a broad range of human activities. This is not only one of its strong

---

comfortable, warm offices. This event is usually held to mark the beginning of a radical change in the relations between major firms and the trade unions in Italy.

points: it is also a potential weakness. It is a strength because it shows that it can be very effective at tackling new and emerging issues in real time, as it did with the technological revolution in the tertiary sector. It is a weakness because it risks looking like a discipline with such a broad range that it loses in terms of depth. But ergonomics is not a discipline with a corpus of notions and with specific tools, for which the huge scope of issues tackled could be detrimental, but a methodology for involving the various kinds of disciplinary knowledge that are necessary for developing on a theme, and as such it only stands to benefit from such a vast array of different experiences.

6.4   Holistic Ergonomics[7] and Classical Ergonomics

What we call "classical" ergonomics refers to the physical model of man, to his measurements, to the means at his disposal and to his physiological and biological limits and may appear to be reductive and unchangeable. As a matter of fact, however, the individual's physical relationship with objects, places and systems is becoming increasingly less decisive, while more and more importance is attributed to the relationship between what is designed and individual and community memories, models of behaviour and emotions.

That is why I am now proposing a new model, one that detracts not one iota from "classical" ergonomics, but opens a window on what I term "holistic ergonomics". What I want to expound here is a more articulated way to go about managing the complexity of human actions and controlling the design of places, products and systems intended to cater for them.

THINKING ABOUT IT

The example I find clearest for explaining this is the mobile telephone. While its dimensions and the ease with which we can put it in our pocket and handle it are certainly important, the real challenge is understanding it and ensuring that it understands us, evaluating the symbolic value that each of us attributes to it and recognising the changes it induces or will induce us to make in our social behaviour. Being easy to handle is of no use if we don't know how to switch it on, if we are afraid of it or if it makes us feel a fool. And these issues are determined by the characteristics of each individual, by the real use we make of it, by how we relate to others, by our habits and behaviour, by our propensity to technology and so on. In all of this the manuals are of precious little use, while a decisive role is played by subjective investigations, surveys about how attractive we find the object, our readiness to venture into uncharted terrain and predictive issues. In other words, we have to observe knowledge, methods of investigation and predictive faculties through a fisheye lens, broadening the package of methods and tools of investigation that we use.

---

[7]The philosophical stance of holism is based on the idea that a system's properties cannot be explained exclusively in terms of its component parts. The word itself, together with its adjective holistic, was coined in the 1920s by Jan Smuts, who defined holism as "the tendency in nature to form wholes that are greater than the sum of the parts through creative evolution".

6.5   The Primacy of Italian Industrial Design: How Come?

Many friends of mine, especially from abroad, have asked me how it was that design in Italy could already started enjoying the development that everyone now acknowledges as long ago as the fifties and sixties, even though the country's production structure was not internationally competitive in those days. Radios were made by Grundig, Philips and Telefunken, scooters did not even exist and gramophones were more or less works of craftsmanship. And yet portable radios and television sets were changed once and for all in those years under the hands of designers like Zanuso and Sapper and the same kind of success was reflected by upholstered furnishings, and that is without even mentioning the Vespa.

Yet the question remains: How come?

I have always tried to provide a logical answer that, in my opinion, illustrates the changeover from technological innovation to innovation of use.

Ergonomics applied to industrial design is particularly active these days in the field of industrial products intended for mass production and/or with advanced technology, both because of the significant role that industrial design has come to play with regard to the development of quality and because of the evolution of the complex relations in which technology, design and the need to cater for human needs are all involved in the creative project. Thinking about how these factors relate to each other led me to identify three characteristic moments in the development of industrial products in Italy: the first was when the engineer's work predominated, the second was when the designer held sway and the third is that of the working group.

- 1st period (until the 1950s)

Technology—Engineers

The project's leadership and issues related to market demand are in the hands of technology and the technologist.

- 2nd period (until now)

Image—Designer

The market now demands quality of performance and quality of form.

- 3rd period (current trend)

Quality—Working Group

The figurehead of the designer/genius is not enough anymore: a design project calls for many different skills.

- 1st period (until the 1950s)

Technology—Engineers

The project's leadership and issues related to market demand are in the hands of technology and the technologist.

- products are simple
- each component fulfils a function
- the design is the work of an engineer
- objects are chosen for their performance
- ergonomics is absent

A first period (which lasted from the beginning of mass production until the 1950s) is characterised by the supremacy of technology and of engineers.

The products made in this period were simple from a standpoint of usage, as each function was fulfilled by a clearly identifiable component. Just think of the structure of the mechanical typewriter, which was strongly influenced and connoted by the levers that controlled the keys. The object's structure described its function unequivocally.

If we look at the example of the evolution of the automobile, we find that in the thirties and forties it was an object that bore all the hallmarks of its technology. That was of course the period when the technical and mechanical innovations were developed that were to transform the car profoundly and give it the characteristics of a mature product. Cars' functional aspects were designed by engineers and then dressed up by the coachworks, specialists who were part designers and part craftsmen. This should not be seen as a value judgement about the results of their work, which were often of high quality, also in terms of their design, but it is interesting to note that the conceptual approach treated technical issues as predominant and those of design and usage as consequential.

Those who bought these products were interested primarily in the performance they could provide and their technological innovations, which were often revolutionary.

In this period, ergonomics, which we can understand as an organic attitude that pays attention to the characteristics of human beings and to their needs, was absent.

- 2nd period (until now)

Image—Designer

The market now demands quality of performance and quality of form.

- products are still quite simple
- designers are charismatic leaders
- designers propose the overall image (the stroke of genius)
- technician put it into practice
- objects are chosen for their design
- ergonomics is an optional extra (an add-on)

The second period, which still lasts today, is characterised by the supremacy of image and of the designer.

Today's products, materials and technologies are still quite simple, so it is easy for them to be mastered by designers, who are specialised in designing an image but not necessarily in the specifics of the various products. Technological issues are considered to be an important feature of the design project, although they are subordinate to the objective of providing products whose formal qualities are unitary and original.

Buyers increasingly often choose on the basis of the quality of a product's image, which actually corresponds very well to new models of lifestyle. This explains why many traditional objects or others with quite a low degree of technological content could be upgraded in Italy with the inventiveness of design, which is also inventiveness applied to new models of use that are more consistent with how society evolves. Just think of the first portable television sets, which broke with the mantra of the television as a status symbol.

THINKING ABOUT IT

Zanuso once told me how he had ventured to design the "Cubo" radio for Brionvega.

A friend of his had brought the idea of the American-style kitchen over from the United State and has founded a firm that he called Homelight, which had built up an extensive chain of shops. One day, he asked Zanuso to make something to sell, to make the most of this opportunity. When Zanuso suggested a portable radio, nobody asked him how many other portable radios he had already designed. That question would have been the first (and the last) if the client had been Grundig, Philips or any of the others. Those firms could not afford to make mistakes and the best guarantee for them was to commission their designs from people who had always done them and would always continue to do them... all of them identical. Zanuso did not start out from the object, but from how its use was evolving and could be theorised: a truly portable object that deserved to be kept on show.

For the technical part, he chose Brion, who was an outsourcing manufacturer, in other words a fully equipped one, but who had no catalogue of his own: the kind of situation that now describes many Chinese manufacturers. Brion evaluated the risk and said he could probably make 1,000 per annum. Everyone knows that they still make 1,000 of them every week to this day.

That was what made Italian entrepreneurship so strong in the sixties!

The Period of Design Enters a Critical Phase

The finished product corresponds less and less to the original idea.

- standards and rules (safety and comfort)
- quality of performance (usability)
- emerging trends (environmentalism and energy saving)
- the limits set by marketing
- sophisticated technology and IT
- specialisation taken to extremes

To simplify, it could be said that where a design project previously started out from the logic of technology, which constituted the object's appeal, in the period of design the project encompassed an idea that combined design, a creative invention and a stroke of genius that obliged the technicians to bend the production technology and methods to the overall aims as proposed, so that the final result would be as close as possible to the original idea, by achieving acceptable compromises in terms of the quality of the object's technology and performance.

It is here that Italian design's great inventiveness and fortune can be found.

Ergonomics started to be introduced at this stage, but as an optional extra to be brought into play towards the end of the design process, to add a further touch of quality that was in any case treated as an accessory.

It is worth noting that this is the model of professional training to which a large proportion of design teaching refers.

In very recent years, the model of organisation that entrusted the development of the mass-produced industrial object to the creativity of designers and its engineering and actual translation into a product to technicians has entered a critical phase because the realisation dawned that a product engineered by technicians ended up corresponding less and less to the synthesis of ingenious image conceived by the artist. This happened because of the advent of a series of increasingly binding factors and the constant increase in the complexity of design and engineering: the standards and rules that govern safety and comfort have become increasingly stringent, increasingly high degrees of performance quality (usability) are now required, important new environmental and energy saving trends have emerged and more and more limits are imposed by marketing, technology and IT. An increasingly high degree of specialisation is also now required, and a new role has come to be played by manufacturers of components that end up exerting a significant influence on how the design idea develops.

At one time, the approach adopted to produce an object entailed one or two people developing every detail of its design project, after which these documents were given to the cheapest and most reliable manufacturer who used them to make the object. In the case of complex mass-produced objects, this model is no longer viable. The technical performance, legal compliance and usability required for producing a system or its component parts have become so specific that they often exceed the entire knowledge accumulated by the ultimate manufacturer, because they call for highly specialised notions and means. As a result, component producers end up not just acting as suppliers in the classical sense of the term, but taking on the role of suppliers of products and proposers of know-how and ideas. Meanwhile, the ultimate producer, who first had the idea for the product and will market it, becomes increasingly a system of design and distribution services whose industrial side is strongly oriented towards assembly.

THINKING ABOUT IT

The fact that complex products have become the sum total of complexities and that specialisation is increasingly extreme hit me clearly when I was working with Fiat, when I realised that even the simplest component was made, designed and often patented by an outsourced supplier. One example was the courtesy light with its three simple functions: on, off and on when the door is open. It could hardly be simpler! And yet very few manufacturers are capable of guaranteeing that the quality of the glass shield will remain unchanged at 80 °C and at −30 °C, that it will always be as clear as crystal, but never fragile and so on.

A design project, then, is oriented by the proposals made by the producer, by technical and legal restrictions, by market requirements and by the demand for quality of use and sensory qualities.

- 3rd period (current trend)

Quality—Working Group

The figurehead of the designer/genius is not enough anymore: a design project calls for many different skills.

- suppliers conduct research, develop, propose and produce
- the brand company assembles
- designers have the following design input:

  - market requirements
  - proposals made by suppliers
  - analysis of qualities of use
  - analysis of sensory qualities

- designers thus receive an often inconsistent body of solutions
- designers transform them into an overall, consistent image using their creativity
- objects are chosen for their usability

This brings us to the third period, which encompasses the trend currently developing and is characterised by quality and by group work.

Users appreciate objects' qualities of use more and more all the time, because they take it for granted that the product will provide them with the technical performance they expect. In fact, unlike what would have happened just twenty or thirty years ago, no buyer of a new car these days would open up the bonnet and start messing around with the engine, because it is now considered to be a closed box, unknown and reliable. The focus nowadays is on how comfortable and attractive the object is how, characteristics that end up guiding our buying decisions. In order to cater for these needs, new models of organisation are being developed in many fields of production (such as automotive, domestic appliances and electronics), which aim to achieve quality, especially in the case of complex mass-produced objects, and propose a design process organised by working groups involving specialists from the various sectors implicated in developing the product and in the various related disciplines. In this respect, increasing importance is being attributed to specialists who study usability and attractiveness. As a result, the application of ergonomics to the design project becomes practically obligatory and not just a check to run on the finished product.

In this context, designers work to transform the various kinds of input, an inconsistent accumulation of these various issues, in an overall consistent image, intervening in the working group with their specific skill, which is their creativity.

It might be thought that this working method would end up impoverishing the design's quality and originality, but that does not happen if the designer is capable of acknowledging all the restrictions, old and new, and working to ensure that they do not act as a brake on the conception, but as a stimulus, orienting his creative abilities to give a sense of unity and originality to what tends to be a motley collection of conditions, so that the final product as a whole is both original and an object of quality.

It is against this backdrop that we in Italy have witnessed an increase on the part of manufacturing firms in interest in products' ergonomic quality. Structures for analysing the usability of hardware and software and university bodies for checking and verifying that products comply with ergonomic specifics have been created. These bodies have hosted the development of techniques of investigation devised specifically to cater for the needs and timeframes set by production industry, both in the field of usability and, more recently, in that of products' sensory qualities, which can be considered the most advanced areas of research into product quality, along with safeguarding the health, physical integrity and well-being of users, the classical field of interest of ergonomics.

This brings us to a point where ergonomics, construed as a strict methodology, meets with design, giving rise to the concept that to work in ergonomics means to design. Because ensuring that places, products and systems become suitable for human beings entails modifying them, and modifying them entails intervening with a project to correct the situation or, preferably, with one of new conception.

But ensuring that objects comply with human needs also entails the object's qualities of form, because it is inconceivable that an object can be considered ergonomically correct if users refuse it because of the image it projects. It is here that we find the link in the chain between ergonomics and the prerogatives of design.

The latest trends today are also exerting increasing pressure to consider the emotive aspects of products (holistic ergonomics) and the commitment to usability for all (Design for All).

Chapter 7
The Built Environment

7.1 Ergonomics and Architecture

From the very start, ergonomics has focused primarily on the workplace: the place where effort is expended and where danger lurks. Yet it did not take long to realise that the problems found in the everyday living environment are not so very different from those of the working environment and that the tools devised for the workplace could also be applied to good effect to everyday life.

THINKING ABOUT IT

Is there any need to ask why it is that the home is significantly more dangerous than the workplace? The statistics are clear! And yet no particularly harmful substances are handled and the environment is familiar, so it ought to be friendly.

There is a reason: the workplace that is the home does not have to comply with standards, rules and laws, it has no specific safety structures, but relies on nothing but common sense, which is often in short supply. How many times have you seen home-made protection guards added to sharp table edges at the height of toddlers' eyes? Or rickety staircases … "we never use them anyway"! These are issues we should be thinking about a lot these days, as working at home becomes increasingly common.

The inclusive design philosophy is more pertinent than ever here, because the realisation has dawned that, both in the workplace and in the places where we live our lives, it is not only right to facilitate everybody: it is also necessary. The fact is that everything should be designed with care these days more than ever before, because the traditional natural buffers that used to enable us to manage our lives by choosing how to organise our physical and social experiences and our relationships are now tending to disappear.

THINKING ABOUT IT

Take how children play, for example: gone are all the trees to climb, the birds' nests to search for and the roads to play in that I remember from my childhood. So artificial situations now have to be created for children to play, with all the problems connected to knowledge of their needs and limits necessary for achieving a human approach to

© Springer Nature Switzerland AG 2019
L. Bandini Buti, *Ask the Right Question*,
https://doi.org/10.1007/978-3-319-96346-4_7

designing, installing and managing play areas. And the same applies to all sorts of different issues, from the food we eat to our holidays (which are also increasingly artificial), our leisure time (all aboard together for a cruise!), the sports we practise and so on.

This is why ergonomics steps in (remembering its original slogan of "adapting work to man") as a discipline suited to the evolution of the modern world: managing complexity.

It is no coincidence that it has apparently become indispensable in high-tech situations (nuclear power stations or the aerospace industry), is applied extensively in the production of highly competitive consumer durables (cars or domestic appliances), has been acknowledged as crucial in the software industry and is now making its way into all schools that deal with design issues.

Despite this, ergonomics is still a rare bird that is seldom seen flying in design projects concerned with town planning and with architectural design in general. Why is this?

I have tried to find an answer to this conundrum and have come to the conclusion that the reason is because many perceive ergonomics to be a discipline related to the dimensions of the human being, so as a source for the anthropometric data that every good designer is capable of applying if he uses a good manual.

It ought to be clear by now that this may be the case of classical ergonomics, but it certainly is not that of the holistic ergonomics that deals with not only the body, but also the mind and the socio-physical environment.

Designing a conception and designing a correction.

The means and tools devised by and for holistic design can be highly effective for identifying situations of potential risk in existing, active buildings and organisations, i.e. in the ones that have already manifested their positive aspects and their defects, where the only possible intervention is one of correction, with all the problems and limits it entails.

But when ergonomics is called into contribute to places and systems that are still in the design phase, things are substantially different, as at this stage the task is to manage concepts and build forecasts rather than analyse material objects, where it is possible to apply cognitive and instrumental analytical techniques.

The fact that it is desirable to intervene when things are still at the level of concepts is confirmed if we remember that real prevention takes place during the design process, ensuring that the situations of difficulty are designed out in good time, rather than waiting for them to crop up in a new structure, but one that needs to be corrected as soon as it is completed.

THINKING ABOUT IT

The first applications of ergonomics in the working environment in Italy were obviously remedial. In those days, the idea of a good design focused on the human being was still in the future. So technicians were sent to do their rounds, taking measurements of noise and pollution that then enabled them to make corrective decisions.

But the time inevitably came when, together with the Director of the Milan Labour Clinic, Nino Grieco, we agreed that real prevention takes place during the design process, when all options are still open.

It was a revolution!

The technicians whose measurements had always guided design culture no longer had anything to measure. All there was of the design of the future was a set of drawings and maybe a drowsy cornfield slumbering in the sun... and that is how the area of design was invaded by people capable of thinking predictively, in terms of models and hypotheses: engineers, architects and designers.

The first step in drawing up an ergonomic design process for the built environment is to introduce the knowledge, means and tools of ergonomics from the very start of that process. This is done by setting up an interdisciplinary working group that includes not only the professionals who will tackle the technical issues, but also others who work with the needs and characteristics of human beings. But guiding a working group made up specialists from different backgrounds is far from straightforward and must comply with the working methods and techniques drawn up by ergonomics in half a century of hands-on experience.

THINKING ABOUT IT

The prospect of the need for alternative working models has been in the air for some time, especially in the field of information technology. Creative work is often done in the West, leaving the 'dirty' work to be done in India or South-East Asia. So it is not enough that the creatives do not get tired or ill or practise absenteeism: they also have to have a stimulating atmosphere. Offices of this kind, such as Google's, sometimes look more like a kindergarten than the editorial desks of a newspaper!

7.2 The Ergonomic Design of the Built Environment

Design that pays due attention to individuals' needs and requirements inevitably calls for a plurality of kinds of expertise, and so of experts, each with his own different tasks, skills and responsibilities: experts in town planning and related legislation, in architecture and engineering, in infrastructures and energy and in human and organisational issues. Unlike the way things were done in the nineteenth century, it is no longer possible these days for a single expert to have all these skills, because the issues in question have become vastly more sophisticated (consider, for example, the technical, psychological and social issues deriving from living in underground environments) and the specialisations necessary have become so differentiated that the design process now involves people who traditionally had nothing to do with construction: psychologists, sociologists, physiologists, doctors in labour medicine etc.

THINKING ABOUT IT

Applying these principles correctly is not enough on its own to guarantee widespread well-being, which is also related to complex socioeconomic factors. Back when I studied, it was nothing unusual to come across the Utopian belief that 'healthy' architecture would make better human beings. We were convinced that the Swedes must be better than us because they had so much vegetation in their cities and efficient services and public transport. When I realised that Sweden had twice as many suicides per capita as us, even though we lived in disastrous cities (in the fifties), with no master plans and no vegetation, I had to think again and become more realistic, more combative and also more cynical.

The correct formula is that good architecture does not necessarily make better human beings, although bad architecture certainly makes people worse.

For projects on a certain scale, the consolidated approach is to piece together an interdisciplinary technical working group, which is considered indispensable for achieving positive results. But giving a working group made up of specialists from different backgrounds an ergonomic orientation is far from easy and must be done using precise working methods.

THINKING ABOUT IT

For example, we cannot and we should never talk about places equipped with efficient light fittings and furnishings that are generically suitable for people (this is the approach adopted by a certain strand of ergonomics that slavishly applies manuals and is proposed by what passes for good technique when it only tackles individual issues one at a time): the right approach is to say that a lighting system is correct only if it is designed as a function of the tasks—and that means all the tasks—that will be done in the area, of the quality and characteristics of the furnishings and the equipment, of the characteristics of the natural lighting, of maintenance and so on.

7.3   Environmental Issues

Great care must be paid to analysing and managing buildings' environmental aspects, since the possibility of running a 'natural' check on the built environment is very slim these days. On the one hand, people demand a high level of wellness in buildings, while on the other the activities carried out in them are becoming increasingly sensitive to critical environmental parameters.

THINKING ABOUT IT

I am old enough to remember when the publisher Mondadori had its head offices scattered around in a series of residential flats that had been adapted for use as offices. Three steps up would take you into the one next-door; there was a bathroom, but only on the floor downstairs and so on. In every room there was usually a 'boss' with one or more secretaries and a typist. The interior designer had provided a window, a heater, some lamps and the curtains. The environment was managed as it would have been at home. If it was hot, you'd open the window a little, but taking care that the typist did not get into a draught, as she was pregnant. Exactly as you would do when managing your home.

But then somebody needed to write a letter in French and the typewriter (and the typist, too) was not suitable. So the text would be sent to another room where all the specialised typists sat together. They might have used pneumatic post to send it. The office organisation became complex and increasingly like that of a workshop.

Mondadori asked Oskar Niemeier to design a new open-space head office outside town, whose interiors would be extremely flexible, but completely controlled and sealed off. It was impossible to open a window or move a curtain. Gone was the environment's 'family' management: the users could not correct anything by opening or closing windows to suit their individual needs, or by varying the local climate (too much sun, the variation in temperature in the course of the day or from hour to hour, individual propensities etc.). It was the designer who had to foresee all the cases of natural lighting, microclimate and mobility, so had to know all the cases that could possibly occur. Not on his own, but assisted by other specialists.

Natural and artificial lighting must be adapted to the activities taking place in the environment and must also be adaptable to the needs of individuals with failing sight (e.g. the elderly). The relationship between natural and artificial lighting and that between the ambient lighting and local workstation lighting must comply with the characteristics and dynamics of the activities taking place there.

The decision to design buildings with plenty of light is often a result of modernist trends more than of real needs. In fact, buildings intended to be used as offices were often traditionally designed to be long and narrow, with plenty of windows, so that all the workstations would have sufficient natural light: the aim was to achieve maximum natural lighting. When IT systems started to make their way into the office, designers realised that using them actually required the opposite, low levels of luminance, because of the contrast between the environment and the field of vision and the risk of reflections on the screen. Many office workers installed spontaneous adaptations, closing the window blinds, if there were any, or sticking posters on the glass.

THINKING ABOUT IT

A building recently completed in Milan to house editorial offices has large continuous windows, but on the southern side it has been fitted with a system of adjustable blinds (brises soleil) to control the light inside the building automatically. This means that the people working in the office cannot see out when the weather is fine, but only when if the sky is cloudy, so they are not happy. J. Nouvel applied the same principle in the Institut du Monde Arabe in Paris in 1987, not to control the environment, but for motives of poetry....

When I realise that this change has taken place, I find myself thinking that today's office buildings should be very different from those of the past. They certainly don't need so many windows, but should be closed to the outside, with smaller sightline 'telescopes' (the people inside should always have cognition of how time is passing outdoors) and windows, even quite big ones, in those rooms where computers are not in continuous use (management offices, meeting rooms, break rooms etc.). This mean that the building should be designed starting from the design of its organisation and of its natural and artificial lighting, which would also, incidentally, enable major energy savings to be made in relation to the need/opportunity to design buildings that are much deeper, so much more compact than the old long and narrow model.

The environment inside the building may be polluted by the processes and activities taking place in it (this kind of pollution is subject to the laws and standards governing health in the workplace), by the materials used (also covered by the law) and by atmospheric factors.

Atmospheric pollution reached dramatic levels in Italy's major cities in the fifties (as it does these days in China). This was mainly caused by emissions from factories and heating systems, which gave off powders and gases without there being any law to restrict them, in fact there was not even any real awareness of the problem. That was when a new colour was created, a very dark grey, which enjoyed a fashionable season or two going by the name of "*fumo di Londra*" (London smoke), since it was reminiscent of the city's fog. After many people had been killed by its infamous smog, London took remedial action and in a relatively short time had an acceptable atmosphere once again, as a result of legislation governing fires and the use of coal. The solution was found to be relatively simple: instead of tens of thousands of chimneys belching out smoke, the city installed technically advanced power stations that generated hot fluids. From that moment on, the issue of air pollution became an important one in the politics of nations, of cities and of individuals' consciences.

7.4   Signs in the City

All public spaces and large-scale complexes can be seen as systems of signage, i.e. as places where the people who frequent them have to be able to find their way around them easily if they are to fulfil their function.

Formal messages

Usage calls for the creation of messages that may be *formal:* this encompasses everything that has been created for the purpose of conveying information (street names and house numbers, signage systems for routing, signage systems for pro- hibitions and obligations, indications of places or services).

THINKING ABOUT IT
The formal messages found in many countries are sometimes very ambiguous. In Tokyo, I am told that the houses are numbered according to the sequence of their construction, something that is not at all helpful for wayfinding. I myself have experience of San José, Costa Rica, where a university's address translates more or less as "the second pavement on the right of the old Coca-Cola factory". Which might not be that bad in itself, except that the factory was demolished ten years ago and the only thing left of it is its place name, which is quite meaningless. This is one of those cases when the much-deprecated rational approach really does function, with its names of neighbourhoods and streets, its house numbers and postcodes.

Informal messages

But messages can also be *informal*. These encompass such things as aspects of architecture and finishes whose appearance induces the general public to associate them naturally to messages about how the spaces are used. A gallery and a portico tell us about walking along them, an open or covered square is a focal point, changes in level in floors communicate a change and aspects of the floor surfaces (materials, textures etc.) can tell us about different environmental qualities (indoors, outdoors), while certain kinds of floor (asphalt, cobblestones, paving slabs etc.) tells us about routing, pedestrian or vehicle zones and so on. Blind people rely to a great extent on such informal messages to recognise places.

Formal signs

Then there are *formal signs*: these are all those objects (signs) that constitute a yardstick in the place, with different meanings according to whether the individual is familiar with the place (so uses his direct memory) or broadly unfamiliar (in which case he uses his memory by association), such as geographical elements that divide or mark the boundary of a territory (rivers, canals, the sea, hills etc.) or distant geographical elements that help us find our way (hills or mountains on the horizon). Similar roles are also played by certain tall human constructions (church towers, skyscrapers, television towers etc.) and lower or smaller buildings that provide points of reference and that need not always be on a large scale (churches, pubs and small monuments etc.).

THINKING ABOUT IT

This is why I appreciate certain signs that architecture has left in many areas of Milan. If we remember that Milan has no rivers, no mountains and no hills that can help us find our way around, then artificial wayfinding aids are more than welcome.

Informal signs

Lastly, our cities are full of *informal signs*. These are all those intangible elements that give places their character and have a different meaning as signage according to whether the individual is familiar with the place (when they have a specific meaning) or broadly unfamiliar (when the meaning is generic). They include differences in lighting in various zones (e.g. exit areas, staircases and lifts, which have brighter lighting in underground carparks), kinds of furnishings (e.g. areas with seating that is typical and characteristic of a waiting area, the use of quality materials in prestigious environments and so on), the calibre of the roads (as an indication of which one has right of way), the presence of vegetation as a landmark and so on.

When elements of signage are managed suitably, they can help make places recognisable (where am I?) and routes identifiable (which way should I go?).

Not everybody perceives the meaning of signs in the same way, because perception depends on the individual's biological, social and cultural characteristics. The differences that abound may be of language (influencing how we understand written messages), of our understanding of codified signs and symbols or of our ability to attribute a meaning to the informal messages typical of the built environment (a capacity that is common among inhabitants of urban cultures). The same also applies to how we use formal signs to recognise places: the general public can understand some of them, because they refer to stereotypes that we recognise regardless of the nature of the specific object (a church, a railway station, a market etc.), while others will only be understood if they have been memorised in advance.

7.5 Signage

As we leave one millennium behind and venture into the new one, Western culture is a culture of communication. Not only because it is so much easier to move around (it's as easy to take a holiday in Bali these days as to go to Viareggio) or because of the worldwide communication web that enables us to speak to the whole world in real time, but also because it impacts on our everyday lives and influences them.

> THINKING ABOUT IT
>
> You only have to venture onto a motorway to realise that the natural message on which we have always based our sense of wayfinding is of no use any more, but can actually get us lost. If we want to go to a town that we can see clearly up there on a hill on the left of the motorway we are driving along, we must not go to the left, as natural logic would tell us, but must follow the road signs slavishly as they invite us to follow a long and winding road that picks its way between advertising hoardings and noise barriers, eventually bringing us to our desired destination.

A poor perception of signs can generate conditions of risk, especially in situations of alarm. It certainly causes anxiety when it does not enable us to obtain the information we want or calls on us to expend mental effort to elaborate its meaning.

> THINKING ABOUT IT
>
> Until quite recently, every Milan street used to have a road sign that told you on which day you were not allowed to park there because the street would be washed on that day. It would read for example "No Parking—Thursday from 0.00 to 6.00", which had to be interpreted, because if you wanted to park in that street on Wednesday evening, you could not leave the car there overnight because it would be towed by the authorities. But as the sign clearly stated "Thursday" you had to elaborate it to understand that "Thursday— 1 = Wednesday". In strictly bureaucratic terms, the sign was correct (0.00 on Thursday is the same as midnight on Wednesday), but it was extremely ambiguous because the word "Thursday" was dominant and did not correspond to the way our mind works naturally.
>
> In many European airports, there are passport gates reserved for "non-Schengen passports", which translated into ordinary parlance means "passports of all foreigners who come from countries outside the European Union and European Economic Area". The sign is bureaucratically correct, but how many Kenyans are certain that this is the correct passport channel for them when they arrive for the first time? And what will happen to the British after Brexit?

What this tells us is that if we want to design a signage or wayfinding system, we have to use suitable means and tools, and the first step is to do what is suggested by the ergonomics manuals, where we can find clear indications about the right sizes for the signs and their lettering if we want to ensure that they are legible, how high they should be off the ground for the information to be comfortably visible at eye level, the right colour contrast to use so that they can be seen for what they are and many other important points.

But they have nothing to say about how the contents should be constructed.

The signage in a built environment may be of pertinence to office buildings, stations, exhibitions and trade fairs, hospitals and a whole host of other kinds of buildings that are expected to be used by a wide variety of people. But the same issues are also relevant to the wayfinding in our city streets, in fact they are vastly more complex. The more varied the users, the more complex the structure and the more occasional and sporadic are the visits people pay to the place, the more their use will take place in situations with the potential to generate anxiety and the greater should be the attention paid to how they are designed. I believe that the highest degree of critical significance is found in large hospitals.

Signage in the built environment

The signage used in the built environment must be able to answer the questions "where am I?" and "which way should I go?". The usual ways of answering these are signposts and written displays, but there are also others.

This information should be conveyed, however, using first and foremost the wayfinding potential of finishes and architectural details, which can send significant messages about orientation, directions and recognisability. Only in those cases where such informal means are incapable of furnishing sufficient explanation should formal signage be relied on to guide people to their destinations.

This has important implications, because it means that the thinking about who is going to use the structure, for what purposes and with what cognition must start at the same time as the idea of the design for the building: it should not be a last-moment add-on.

THINKING ABOUT IT

Here's an anecdote. At the beginning of the last century in via Farini 63, in Milan, a shopkeeper had the fine idea to create a balcony above his store by composing the wording "G. Rossi, Conserve alimentari" (G. Rossi, Grocery Preserves) in concrete Art Nouveau lettering, making a fine statement of confidence that he expected his business to last for a very long time!

How many times have I seen a fine brass nameplate set in the wall next to the door of an office bearing the name of the owner, but covered over with a scrap of paper attached with sticky tape because nobody thought that mobility is a typical feature of our day and age. Maybe a little common sense would have helped them realise it.

The first instinct that a designer may have when called on to create a wayfinding system in a complex place is to think of what signs to install. The result is often an over-abundance of pointless information.

THINKING ABOUT IT

In a small town in Italy's region of Emilia, located near the point where two important motorways meet, for example, I have seen direction signs at some road junctions that pointed the way towards the A1 motorway (or sometimes towards Bologna, Milan or Parma), while at other junctions they pointed the way towards the A15 motorway (or towards La Spezia) and at other junctions again they just pointed the way towards "autostrade" (motorways). For me, the message was crystal clear: there were two different direction for the A1 and the A15, but at some points they coincided.

But that's not at all how it is!

in the end, I found the entrance to the A1 motorway. I found that it was the same as the entrance for the A15: the two motorways split after the tollbooth. The sign system has led me uselessly to raise my level of concentration, making me believe something that was not the case: the only correct sign was the one that indicated nothing but "autostrade".

I am almost sure that the root of this confusion is the fact that two or more authorities installed the signage for which they were responsible, each following its own logic and probably at different times. One thing is certain, in any case: nobody had ever bothered to develop a communication design that ought to be the only correct way to answer the simple question that a driver asks himself—"which road should I take to go to…?"—and that calls for the installation of the minimum number of information points, but ensures that they are co-ordinated, effective and short. And that tells me that it is not enough to have good graphic designers to get good information: you need to have decision-makers who think.

Then there are the manuals that tell you what size you should make your letters, your signs and so on. That's all well and good, but how do you construct the contents? Very little is ever said about this or it is just taken for granted.

Yet that is what we shall try to do.

THINKING ABOUT IT

I once had the opportunity to work with my colleague, the architect Franco De Nigris, on developing the signage system inside the head office of Italy's major daily newspaper, *il Corriere della Sera*, in Milan's via Solferino. We realised that a great deal of information is published about the most appropriate use of fonts, their legibility as a function of distance, the shape of signs and the colour of the background and the lettering… but little or nothing about their contents.

This gave us the chance to develop a methodology that enabled us to identify three clear main issues to be considered when designing a signage system: what the subject of the signage is, where the signs will be located and how the information is to be represented.

When we go about defining the contents and graphics of an information system in a place in the built environment, the best way is to proceed with a sequence of working phases: the classification of the places, the definition of the routing and the identification of nodal points. With this information in hand, you can then proceed to create the wayfinding system and run a first check using simple, inexpensive means, after which you will have all the elements you need for the actual graphic design process.

Identifying and setting limits

The first thing we need to know when defining an effective, efficient wayfinding system is the identification of the places that people will seek out as destinations or as nodal points: entrances of various kinds (pedestrian or vehicle), horizontal channels of communication (corridors), vertical channels of communication (stairwells, lifts and escalators), the constituent elements into which the building can be broken down, i.e. homogeneous units such as blocks of the building (e.g. the wings of a hospital), departments with homogeneous usages and all the areas and the services related to production (in industrial areas) or the building's management.

The areas thus identified often do not coincide with clearly defined physical spaces. An open space department may be made up of zones that are structurally identical, but quite different in terms of how they relate to the public or of other parameters that guide the decisions about signage.

Names

Signage must use place names that are either familiar or can be learned and are capable of identifying destinations clearly. The fact is that the same destination is often defined in more ways than one. In hospitals with multiple wings and buildings, for example, it is quite common to find that one department is known both by the name of the building it is housed in (e.g. "Queen Margherita Wing") and also by its content, i.e. by the medical speciality it houses, and this can generate confusion. In such cases, one name should be chosen and used exclusively.

> THINKING ABOUT IT
>
> Other names derive from previous events that nobody remembers any more today. The lecture theatres in one area in a university I know are called "CT" because they are housed in what used to be factory buildings belonging to a firm called "Ceretti e Tanfani". But the lecture theatres in the building next door are called "CS", because they are accessed through an entrance from via Cosenz. This creates no difficulty for people who frequent the campus every day, but it can be a major issue for the occasional visitor.

At the *Corriere della Sera,*[1] everyone identified the buildings by the street onto which their main doors opened (Via Solferino, Via San Marco, Via Montebello and Via Moscova).

We found that the identification of these entrances was correct, because the names chosen must be:

- *meaningful*: agree with the idea that the people using them have of the object;
- *memorable*: straightforward and easy to remember and note down;
- *transmittable*: easy to transmit by word of mouth, also considering phonetic uncertainties;
- *unequivocal*: there must be no chance of confusion between the names.

Like every design project, a signage project should start by asking "who?", i.e. by identifying the people who for any reason will spend time in the place. They will certainly have different degrees of cognition, different habits and different objectives.

---

[1]Translator's note: the *Corriere della Sera* is a leading Italian daily newspaper, published in the country's business capital, Milan, and traditionally expressing the point of view of the northern business community.

– *Operatives*

These are the people who conduct their activities in the structure on a continuous basis. They have substantially standard characteristics and can be considered to have specific acquired knowledge, the possibility to access information and have often benefitted from training of a formal kind (courses, meetings and events) or informal in nature (knowledge picked up from colleagues). In addition, as they belong to the structure, it is possible to set rules for them (for example, no parking in certain areas).

– *Habitual users*

These are people who visit the structure frequently for any reason whatsoever. They are for example the clients of a bank, the people who park in an underground carpark and so on. They have the common characteristic of having specific acquired knowledge that facilitates them when they use the structure.

– *Occasional users*

These are people who use the structure seldom or for the first time. They are for example patients at the emergency room, the relatives of patients in a hospital and so on. They have the common characteristic of having no specific knowledge, but we can consider that they have the general level of knowledge that is shared by the large categories of users to whom they belong (for example, everyone who drives knows the highway code and the meaning of road signs).

– *Other categories*

When developing the design for the flows of movement inside the structure, we should always consider what particular situations may arise in relation to it that do not fall under any general heading.

One quite common case for which allowance must be made is the presence of important guests or visitors. Another frequent case is that of access for visiting school groups.

7.6   Identifying the Nodal Points

Nodal points are places where it is necessary or opportune to provide wayfinding.

By virtue of their vocation, nodal points are *entrances* (the ones leading in from external pedestrian or vehicle routes and the ones inside a structure that provide access to its individual units), *horizontal channels of communication* (the points where routes meet junctions, crossways and branches), *vertical channels of communication* (points of access to staircases and lifts) and *meeting points* (the places where people gather together in case of a security alarm, places where people arrive and leave and goods are loaded and unloaded and other places typical of the kind of structure under study, such as the ticket office in a theatre or cinema, waiting rooms in a doctor's surgery etc.). Nodal points are by definition the places where people are uncertain and get lost. This should be remembered and they must be defined with care.

The information compiled by this stage will enable the designer to develop a fully-fledged signage system with articulations in various forms of communication.

The various kinds of information to be provided should be furnished on the following families of signs:

- *Maps for general orientation*, necessary above all in complex structures;
- *Signage for horizontal channels of communications*, showing the directions of roads, corridors etc.;
- *Signage for vertical channels of communication*, showing where staircases, escalators, lifts and ramps lead;
- *Identification of places*, i.e. naming the place where you are or which you access through an entrance.

Just how effective this signage is can be appraised by discussing it with experts and gathering the impressions and comments of people representative of the different categories of users. Observation of how users behave when they acquire information can be a very effective way to gather such knowledge.

The buyer and the user

For the designer, the producer and the sales staff, it is important to know who will make the decision to buy the product or system to be produced, because the attitude to adopt and the resources employed by a person buying for himself are nearly always very different from those employed by a buyer who is buying on behalf of others.

When the buyer and the user are the same person, the mechanism of analysis used to adapt the object to the user's needs may be very sophisticated.

For example, how many even quite subtle things do we consider before we buy a new car? The cost, certainly, its reliability and the after-sales service, but also and above all how well it caters for how we intend to use it on an everyday basis (commuting to the office) and occasionally (going to the seaside on Saturday).

The producer gets immediate feed-back about how well his product caters for the market's requirements (either it sells or it does not sell) and will do everything to adapt to it, so as to improve his product's market penetration. Just look how many often pointless gadgets clutter up our cars, at least on the driver's side, because he is the one who buys the car. The passenger does not even have a footrest: he did not buy the car!

When the buyer and the user are not the same person, the way that the object is adapted to the individual user's needs follows a fundamentally different route.

If you take a train, you have no choice but to use the carriage that arrives at the platform, however comfortable or uncomfortable it may be: you have no chance to influence the quality of the product. At school, you are the one who adapts to the desk that somebody else has chosen for you. The principle of feedback does not function here: the manufacturer has nothing to gain directly from improving his product.

In some virtuous cases, the firm that produces goods or manages services may adopt a policy of taking steps that are oriented towards man and his needs (a Design for All oriented firm), partly because this approach is associated with the desire to appear to be a virtuous firm that keeps abreast of developments. In this case, the techniques of investigation typical of the "Ask the Right Question" approach will be adopted already at the design stage.

But if the products are bought by a procurements office, what parameters of appraisal does it use? The end user will certainly have no way of influencing what is bought. I don't even want to consider the nefarious mechanisms of personal advantage, but what tools does the procurements manager have to enable him to make his choices?

This illustrates the importance of developing a system for disseminating awareness of the characteristics of how the object or system is used and its qualities, by means of such vehicles as a Quality Label guaranteed by serious, accredited third-party bodies and authorities.

Part III
A Practical Application

Chapter 8
Active Ageing

Ageing is the only method we have found so far for living longer.

Most of us have known people whose capacities have undergone drastic change at some stage in their lives. Sometimes it is a traumatic experience, the result of an accident or an operation, while in other cases it is a more gradual process brought about by ageing. The simple process of ageing is strange, as I know from personal experience: for a long time you feel as though nothing has changed, or that the changes that have taken place have no influence, then all of a sudden you realise that so much has changed. All it takes is a minor accident, a moment's distraction or a comparison.

And you will certainly have noticed that these people generally want to stay living in their own homes. Your home is where your heart is, with your affections and your memories: it is full of signs that you alone can see, because they are signs that you left yourself. The nail where you once hung the painting that you took down because you had gone off it, but the nail is still there. You are the only one who sees it. And the mark you made when you rested the ladder against the wall. I think that staying in your own home is something that everybody wants.

Being happy to go back home or to stay there: "I'm going home: I still feel at home there".

In reality, though, the person we are talking about and his surroundings have changed. I'm not just talking about major changes (such as if he cannot walk any more), but also about minor ones (he has difficulty getting up out of a chair if he has nothing to push against, or he gets forgetful and so on). His home is often not such a welcoming place any more, in terms not so much and not only of getting around, but also of its social climate, how it impacts on his relations. His family has a life of its own to live (which is also changing) and there is no guarantee that there is still a significant place in it for him. So he gets a carer who helps him with all his material needs, but he risks becoming an outsider in his own home, so he shuts himself away in his bedroom. Maybe it would be better for him to go into a care home, where they know how to look after him, treat him and feed him, and where he can chat and remember the days that were his good old days because he was much younger.

© Springer Nature Switzerland AG 2019
L. Bandini Buti, *Ask the Right Question*,
https://doi.org/10.1007/978-3-319-96346-4_8

Then there are holidays, when you stay in a hotel or a spa or go on a cruise. They are also situations when you are not at home, but you'd like to feel welcome.

So there are times when you may feel better away from home than at home: "I feel I have been made welcome".

When you build a new house, it is certainly hard to think about the future, since you already have enough problems for today: the decisions you have to make, your mortgage, the move and all the rest. But what we notice is that it is the family that is mobile: children are born, grow up and fly the nest and we all eventually die. The house remains immobile.

For every tiny alteration, you have to start demolishing, rebuilding, adapting, throwing stuff away and buying other stuff. Why is it that life is elastic, but the home is not? In the working world, offices have become elastic in every respect, both physical and in terms of the systems that make them function. Offices have changed but our houses have not!

Why don't we think of an 'elastic house' when we still have time and when adaptations would be cheap and affordable, instead of waiting and having to demolish?

I know why! Because we are superstitious. "I am young and have a good job: why should I worry about when I'll be old and creaky?" But that's such a big mistake! Adaptation is not a matter of coping with a disability, but of the way our lives flow: it should not be for a special event, but for every day.

It's better to be ready: "man changes, so a house can also change".

THINKING ABOUT IT

A school teacher friend of mine was once asked to teach at the middle school that had been established in the Milan institute for the blind as a policy of integration. Invited to a welcome dinner by a couple of blind teachers, she told me all about it. Sitting in a deep armchair in a room that was almost completely in the dark, she heard the couple as they went about preparing dinner: "pass me the salt...", "another couple of minutes, then we'll add the onion...", there was much clatter of cooking implements, all absolutely in the dark. She was the one who felt different and out of place, an intruder.

That's what happens if you go to a 'Dinner in the Dark', where the blind people who accompany you are perfectly at ease and you are not. They prepare your coffee and give you the right change, but you didn't even know that the coins have differentiated tactile values (as an aside: I often wonder how the Americans manage with their greenbacks, whose values are different, while the formats are all the same). Some people cannot manage and leave before the dinner is over.

Incidentally, I prefer the word 'blind' to 'visually impaired' and I'll try to explain why.

The trend to take pains with being politically correct has introduced a series of euphemisms into our language, such as 'visually impaired', 'differently able' and other rather pitiful, saccharine-sweet circumlocutions. I am Italian (it's a fact), I am male (another fact) and I am short (another fact): I am not 'differently tall'.

To be 'blind' is a fact. 'Visually impaired' is an impairment: the term focuses on telling us that somebody has something missing, so is not 'complete'. It's as though I were to talk about a women as a 'non-male', which is indisputably true, but gives the impression that she could be a male, but is a woman because she is not perfect!

8.1   The '*Fatto Apposta*' Project[1]

A few years ago, the local health unit in Vicenza informed the small and medium-sized enterprise association with responsibility for the city and its province, Confartigianato Vicenza, that it did not have the resources it needed to house all the non-self-sufficient elderly people in the city and asked for help to enable them "to go back home content".

In actual fact, nearly all elderly people, as well as those who have had a major accident or operation, need a home that is adapted to their particular requirements. The alterations may be minor or major, but they call for special design attention.

THINKING ABOUT IT

What kind of tap is the right one for a person who has difficulty manipulating things with his hands or cannot exert much force with them? How can an installer or a plumber decide? Is a tap that turns on and off with a screw motion the best one? But the turning action may be a challenge for many... and what about the grip? Should it have three or four very obvious spokes, or a minimalist cylinder with no gripping surfaces, like the ones that so many architects are so fond of? Or would a lever be better? But the lever is not very easy for almost everyone to use. It's easy to have it either all on or all off (just push the lever right up or right down), but fine adjustment calls for the user to dose the effort carefully, maybe by using a spot of ingenuity (such as by moving only the tip or the base of the lever). It is no coincidence that taps in hospitals have a special format with a wide range, so that they can also be used with the elbows.

Then there are taps that are activated by a sensor, which usually have to be accompanied by a note that tells people how to use them (nobody has yet dared to give them a radically updated shape, because everyone is afraid that the market might refuse to accept it).

There is certainly a correct solution, but the plumber (and he is not the only one) does not have the knowledge to make a conscious decision, so more often than not he will rely on his supplier, who will certainly give him an expensive product that he knows will match with the sanitary fittings, which are always a little conservative.

Confartigianato answered by organising training courses for all the hierarchy involved in the design process: those doing the design work (architects, engineers and surveyors), healthcare workers (social service workers and doctors), builders and plant installers and the specialised associations representing the end users. All of them together in one lecture theatre, because the learning process should not be just vertical, the ex-cathedra input of a lecturer imparting his knowledge, but also horizontal, between different stakeholders who often know nothing about each other.

So the lecturers found themselves facing a very heterogeneous assembly that was far from easy to satisfy. If you spoke about the need to gather subjective information, the architects would say that they didn't need you to tell them, since that was what they had always done, while others thought they had done it and others again believed that they already knew everything without the need to make

---

[1]Translator's note: "Fatto Apposta" translates literally as "Made on Purpose", but its usage is more closely related to the principle of "Made to Measure".

so much fuss. One person claimed that, as he had an aunt with hip problems, he knew what he had to do to make everything easily useable for everyone. As though his aunt was some kind of universal prototype!

With such a varied audience, the organisers decided it was out of the question to use standard learning methods, lessons, slides and notes. The lecturers needed to use a language that would cut across the board of the participants' different levels of training, of information and of interests, also considering that they were not exactly school children, but adults and mature professionals.

The method developed was based more on uncertainties than on certainties, obliging participants to identify the issues and to find the responses that would then guide the solutions. In a nutshell, this was the Design for All approach applied to the complexity of human diversity for the purpose of achieving and communicating an inclusive and participatory design process. To this approach, developed by Avril Accolla and myself, we gave the name 'Ask the Right Question'.[2]

THINKING ABOUT IT

The usual way to go about altering a flat to make it suitable for an individual who comes out of hospital with reduced motor functionality is to apply the entrenched rules for a house for a person with disabilities: do away with the steps and install ramps, slopes and grab rails. That kind of design will certainly be generic and reassuring for anyone who does not want to think about it too much, but it will equally certainly be unimaginative or even wrong. A serious designer should ask questions about what the individual can do, how his condition is likely to evolve, his enthusiasm for life and desire to react (also in terms of what he could and used to do before and can no longer do now), with whom he lives and their habits and propensity to adapt to the changes etc. The answers, which we need to source from the people who know, will guide the design process, which should always aim to be creative.

Design for All is design for human diversity, social inclusion and equality.[3] It is a way of tackling design processes and highlights the fact that they can be both ethical and business-oriented.

THINKING ABOUT IT

Here's an example: imagine devices that would help people get around, not products that are immediately classifiable as wheelchairs for people with disabilities, but pleasant, well-designed products that target everybody's needs. They would certainly be a boon in many places, such as museums, trade fairs and other large infrastructures, so could be produced in numbers large enough to be good business. Good business for the manufacturers, but also for the people using them, since the prices would be typical of mass production and not of specialised products.

---

[2]The method was presented by A. Accolla (Tongji University, Arts and Media College, Shanghai, China PRC) and L. Bandini Buti (Milan Polytechnic School of Design, Milan, Italy) at the First International Conference on Design for Inclusion, held in Orlando, Florida, in the framework of AHFE 2016, with a paper entitled *Ask Yourself the Right Question. To know and understand the beauty of Human Diversity it is the first design step: a Design for All structured and autopoietic tool*.

[3]EIDD Stockholm Declaration 2004 ©.

Human diversity generates a complex, continuously changing society. This means that designers and the design process have an enormous social, environmental and economic responsibility. That is the challenge faced by Design for All. 'Ask the right question' could mark a turning point.

In areas where inertia is very strong, for example, such as caring for and managing the elderly, this method could replace the usual approach, which is often based on medical data and on long-established, reassuring responses that, however, inhibit future developments and innovation. This approach should not be restricted to obvious cases of disability, but should also embrace all the situations we encounter in our lives. Is a tourist who visits yet another museum disabled or not? He may well be, because he is tired. And what about a person who gets lost while wandering through the labyrinth of a major hospital and is also suffering anxiety because of the news he is expecting to receive? He also needs to feel welcomed and to benefit from clear, reassuring places and routing.

8.2   Active Ageing

There is no need to make a point here of reiterating that the world's population is ageing. The European Union adopted the issue when it decided that 2012 would be the European Year of Active Ageing and published a specific document[4] which I shall mine here for some interesting data.

"[T]he large cohorts born in the late 1940s and the 1950s are now reaching retirement age [...] the total working-age population (15–64 year-olds) is set to fall by 20.8 million from 2005 to 2030 as the baby-boom cohorts retire. [...] the number of elderly people is increasing rapidly. The number of people aged 80+ is set to increase by 57.1% between 2010 and 2030 (1). This will mean 12.6 million more people aged 80+ in Europe [...]

"Demographic change can be successfully tackled through a positive approach that focuses on the potentials of the older age groups. The concept of active ageing is at the heart of this positive response to demographic change, which is essential to preserve solidarity between generations [...]

"Active ageing [...] means: [...] enabling both women and men to keep in good health and to live independently as they grow older, thanks to a life-course approach to healthy ageing combined with adapted housing and local environments that allow elderly people to remain in their own homes as long as possible. [...]

"Active ageing is the basis for solidarity between generations—a goal of the EU enshrined in Article 3 of the Lisbon Treaty. It means that older people can take charge of their own lives and contribute to society—and allows more to be done for those elderly people who depend most on the support of others."

---

[4]*The EU Contribution to Active Ageing and Solidarity between Generations*, Directorate General for Employment, Social Affairs and Inclusion, Unit D. 3, November 2012. The document is available for download at http://ec.europa.eu/social/main.jsp?langId=en&catId=89&newsId=1632&furtherNews=yes.

8.3   A Methodology: What and How

Why not design for all ... including people with disabilities?

The project to build or adapt homes where elderly people can live out their lives contentedly, whether alone, with their families or in communities, must cater for each individual's needs, because all those individuals are different from one another, in terms not just of their physiological and sensory characteristics and capacities, but also and primarily of their lifestyles, aspirations, needs, wishes and dreams.

> THINKING ABOUT IT
>
> Some elderly people living in a care home were questioned during a design seminar. The outcome was a cross-section of their world that was very different from the idea of the 'scrapheap of society'. The researchers discovered the heritage of knowledge and memories that many of the elderly residents have (a 90-year-old lady told me "it's true that I never married, but I guarantee that I lived my life to the full: I also worked with Fellini". I did not ask her what she meant when she said she had "lived her life to the full", but her eyes said it all). In Romagna, a bicycle is far more than a means of locomotion, but on that occasion we discovered that the bicycle should be redesigned for all those elderly ladies who do not want to stop going to the market on their bikes, but do not feel so safe doing so any more. And it would be a very promising line of business if the bicycles were not made 'for people with disabilities', but 'for people who refuse to make do'.

The activities of 'asking the right question' and 'finding the answer' are particularly well suited to a project for active ageing, because they are oriented towards finding the answers from everyone who can furnish knowledge about the issue, regardless of the education, the kind of language and the interests of the people in question. In fact, there is no way that such a project can avoid involving not only the elderly people themselves in the decisions to be made, but also those who live with them, their doctors and other health personnel and the technicians who know all about the plant systems, as well as the designers and architects in the strict sense of the terms.

Approaching it in this way and using the "Ask the Right Question' methodology, the issue of the habitat for active ageing was tackled in the framework of the 'Fatto Apposta®' project organised by Confartigianato Vicenza in 2013–2014.[5]

'Ask the Right Question' offers a new approach to the issue of enabling the many different stakeholders to take part in a design project, which was articulated in three sections:

---

[5]*Fatto apposta—progetto per l'abitare del futuro*, Confartigianato Vicenza, Vicenza 2014.

(A) Going back home

Feeling at home when I'm at home.

(B) Feeling at home when you are away from home

I feel I have been made welcome

This applies to all the situations where people stay long-term or short-term in community homes or leisure locations or in specialised structures. Elderly people should not be considered to be some sort of standard human beings whose only defining characteristic is that they are old: they are individuals who remember a past that may still be a source of values and who have affections and memories that deserve to be respected.

(C) It's better to be ready

Man changes, so a house can also change.

This applies to all those people who are thinking of getting a new home where they intend to live for a long time. The family is mobile: we are born, we die, we get married, we have children, we leave home etc. But the house remains immobile: it does not change, except at very high cost and with much disturbance. This is very much the case in Italy, where the house is stable (both in terms of its structure and of its durability), less in other places where it is less durable (made of wood and with a relatively short life cycle). But every home can be designed so that it can be adapted in future to suit new needs without too much cost or disturbance.

8.4 Going Back Home

I still feel at home there.

This applies to anyone who has to adapt an existing house to new needs, which may be traumatic, like going back home after an important operation, or gradual, like ageing or the entirely straightforward process of the evolution of the family when a new child is born.

- **When**? *When something has changed.*

When you go back home after a disabling event, such as an accident, an operation or an illness.

- **Why?** *Because going back home may be difficult.*

The individual's motor, sensory and/or cognitive capacities are changed or reduced. The consequences are always traumatic. The individual is, or feels, impoverished in terms of his quality of life, an experience that is often quite unexpected and violent. The house to which he returns after the event will almost certainly have to be adapted to his changed personal conditions.

- **What?** *A house for me, but also for others.*

The changes made to the environment must make life easier for the individual in question without making it difficult for those who share the same home with him (for example, by treating the home as though it were a hospital), because the risk is that family relations might deteriorate and the cause might be identified as the presence of the individual in need. The solution is to make the environment as accessible as possible to his new needs, while at the same time focusing on keeping or making it familiar and positive.

If the home was originally designed to make potential alterations possible (applying the principle of 'it's better to be ready'), the alterations will be relatively simple, since there will be no major technical obstacles: it will just be a matter of modifying spaces and fittings that were originally devised for general situations, so as to suit them to the needs of a specific individual and his lifestyle.

- **Who?** *Who can help me?*

The work done by specialists is bound to target the individual and his pathology, which is certainly well-known and obvious, just as its probable evolution may also be well-known and obvious. The individual's doctor may be able to offer useful assistance and must in any case be consulted from the very start.

- **Ask the right question** *How can I understand?*

You have to ask the right question, but you also have to understand whether your own skills alone will be enough, or whether you also need to call in someone else who has the skills you need. The 'right question' should be addressed directly to the individual (if possible) and to those who live with him and should be compared to the real situation of the built environment.

The purpose of asking the 'right question' is not just to facilitate operational decisions (such as designing, what to use etc.), but primarily to enable the designer to get a hands-on impression of the specifics of each situation. So 'right questions' should also be asked even if you see no immediate design prospects. In other words, the purpose of the questions is not only to enable the designer to understand what sanitary fittings to choose, for example, but also what the right house is and might be like in future.

***

When an important change has taken place in an individual's functional capacities, whether sudden (such as an operation or an accident) or gradual (a developing illness or ageing), the aim is nearly always for the individual in question to be able to go back home, to the place that is inhabited by his memories and affections. But that return home will always be a traumatic experience, awakening easy comparisons between the before (happiness) and the after (resignation).

Many things that he had never even noticed before may now become restrictions: the height of the worktop in the kitchen, the space where he can put his legs underneath it, the height of his bed from the floor and so on.

The house needs to be adapted.

But how? One thing is certain: nobody wants to live in a branch of a hospital and, whenever possible, the home should keep its reassuring family atmosphere. It should certainly enable basic activities and those that give meaning to life to be carried out in the best possible way, but it should also be predictive, predisposed to make due allowance for expected changes and developments that may only be potential.

But the individual who 'goes back home' also has a social life with his family and/or friends. If his family feels obliged to change its lifestyle for the worse, its members will feel they have been mistreated and there is a risk that they will end up 'making him pay'. So the house must also be good for them. That is the task of the architect or designer, who has to gather information by 'asking the right questions'. That task involves getting to know the individual (**getting to know him/her**), getting to know the others who live and/or interact with him (**getting to know the others**) and analysing the environment, so as to understand its potential: what has to/can be changed and what can be kept unchanged (**getting to know the place**).

THINKING ABOUT IT

'Going back home' is something that concerns specific individuals who once inhabited the place in question, gave it meaning and accumulated their stories and memories there, but who now go back there with the limitations imposed by their changed conditions. We can learn about these limitations, because they do not refer to probable but as yet unknown situations, the sort of thing that we might encounter when discussing the issue of 'it's better to be ready', or to a range of problems that may be definable, but generic, such as the ones we might encounter in a community structure. What we have, instead, is a real-life situation as it is here and now and a more or less predictable near future. We are not dealing with an unknown and undefinable 'person with disabilities', but with John Smith, whom we can get to know very well.

(A) Getting to Know Him/Her

Gathering information about the individuals who need changes to be made

The most important source of information when getting to know an individual is found in the various kinds of subjective investigation described in the literature, which should certainly be used with the individual himself (who will probably respond with a vision of hope or of delusion) and with his close family and friends, as well as, in certain circumstances, with the healthcare workers who know him. None of the versions found will provide the absolute truth, but by comparing them the researcher will probably be able to piece together a more complete and articulated vision of the individual and his needs.

(a) The individual's needs

These are what an individual must be able to do if he is to have an acceptable quality of life.

They cover such things as independence in eating and hygiene, mobility, the management of free time and communicating with others, either directly or through intermediaries. There are basically five needs and they exist in a hierarchy of importance that goes from the most basic to the highest levels.

These are physiological needs (survival), the need to be safe and secure (protection), the need for affection (a sense of belonging, love), the need for esteem (personal consideration) and lastly the need for a sense of achievement (of your own potential and your aspirations).

QUESTIONS TO ASK THE INDIVIDUAL AND OTHERS

- What were your needs in the past? (this encompasses the ones that everyone lists when leading an ordinary life, how they have been catered for and how they can still be today);
- What are your new needs? (this encompasses the ones generated by the individual's new condition, such as diet, medical treatment, rehabilitation exercises etc.) and the new problems they cause.

WHY?

- To get to know the characteristics of the structures and/or objects used in the individual's normal everyday activities (in the kitchen, the bathroom and so on) and for whom (for himself or also for others);
- To understand how these activities can continue and what others may be added to the list;
- To understand what can be used, what can be reused with alterations and what has to be replaced.

THINKING ABOUT IT

The architect or designer may tend to focus all his attention on the individual with disabilities and so neglect what others need. Let's take the kitchen, for example. It's almost automatic to think that a good design for going back home would include making a kitchen for a person with disabilities: low worktops, space under them for wheelchair access and so on. But did the individual ever cook before? Maybe not. So a kitchen for a person with disabilities may actually be a hindrance to everyone else! The right thing is to understand whether the individual always used to cook and will be able to continue doing so if he has what he needs, or whether he only used to cook something occasionally (prepare a coffee, heat something up and maybe fry an egg), or whether he never used the kitchen at all. It is only once you know this that you can make the right decision: a specialised kitchen, a kitchen with a specialised corner, or an ordinary kitchen.

Luckily, these days there are kitchens for everyone, with or without disabilities, that solve the issue brilliantly.

(b) The individual's habits

These are the issues of lifestyle that the individual applies in his everyday life and social relations. They concern how he relates to things, to other people and to his family. They also concern the characteristics and qualities of his activities and of his behaviour, as well as his personal preferences in general.

QUESTIONS TO ASK THE INDIVIDUAL

- What were your old habits, the ones we should think of as entrenched?
- What might become new habits, mostly concerning your awareness that there are some things that you will probably not be able to do any more?

WHY?

- To get to know the things that are materially indispensable for preserving his habits (books, music, memories, minor obsessions etc.);
- To understand whether these things can be strengthened, improved or highlighted;
- To get to know how much can be omitted or avoided (or abolished) for reasons of space without it becoming a traumatic experience.

THINKING ABOUT IT

It is dangerous to think of elderly people as no more than stereotypes, in other words as people with problems to which design has to provide the best answer. But the people you will come face to face with often remember their past not so much with nostalgia as with pride: "I was the only carpenter capable of making a double dovetail joint", "I used to travel a lot, but now I can rest". And what about all those 'little old men' who once played important parts in society and have a heritage of knowledge that may be a bit dated, but is still very strong? With a touch of humour, we could say that today's old men are not the same as the genuine article of the old days: they were really little old men. These days they go on a cruise to the Caribbean!

At one time, old age was seen as a source of wisdom. People would pay heed to an old peasant, who knew from experience whether it was better to prune a vine today or wait a little longer. These days nobody pays attention to that kind of experience any more: it's been replaced by science. I don't know whether this is really progress or whether we are the poorer for it.

I suppose people will just say that I am a little old man myself!

(c) The individual's new limitations

These are the objective limitations to the individual's abilities (motor, perceptive and/or sensory) that were already there or that have now come about, or that were already there and have now become more marked. The main source of information for this is the individual's healthcare worker, but the individual himself can also furnish his own perception of his condition.

QUESTIONS TO ASK THE INDIVIDUAL AND HEALTHCARE AND SOCIAL STAFF

- What, if any, limitations were there on your hearing, sight, speech, manual dexterity, ability to walk, memory and cognition?

WHY?

The aim here is to get to know what the individual really needs in order to be able to exercise his abilities, what the other members of his family unit need and so on (i.e. to avoid converting the home to make it look like a hospital!);

- To get to know what limitations, if any, the individual has;
- To understand what steps are indispensable/useful for tackling those limitations;
- To understand what can be used, what can be reused with alterations and what has to be replaced.

(d) The individual's aspirations

These are the objectives that the individual would like to achieve in future. Since individuals are all different, these too may be of all kinds, concerning such things as physical activities (sport, exercise…), intellectual activities (reading, writing, making music or listening to it…), working on hobbies, using leisure time at home or outside the home, looking after others (children, animals…) or working (manual work, working at the computer, voluntary work…).

QUESTIONS TO ASK THE INDIVIDUAL AND OTHERS

- What did you aspire to in the past? (The aim here is to get to know about his activities or the aspirations he already achieved);
- What new aspirations do you have now? (The aim here is also to investigate his awareness of his current condition and to what extent he is pro-active).

WHY?

- To get to know what tools and environments he would need to achieve his new aspirations;
- To understand how much of what already exists should be kept;
- To understand how much of what already exists can be suitably adapted;
- To understand what new tools and environments need to be provided for.

THINKING ABOUT IT

At the price of sounding like an unreformed romantic, I cannot help remembering that the smaller communities that used to exist before the Industrial Revolution contributed to preserving roles and relationships. Everyone knew everyone else and had probably shared experiences with them. People would meet in the local inn or village hall, places where they would compete with each other, share their stories and experience love.

These days we are more likely to make friends with a blogger who lives in Hong Kong than with the family that lives on the other side of the landing. Relationships have moved from physical to virtual. Children do not rush off in gangs to steal unripe fruit off the trees any more (it was never about the fruit anyway, but about breaking the rules), so we need to create places like playgrounds. Architects and designers have the serious (and exciting) task of transforming a shopping centre, for example, into a place that is not just for shopping, but primarily for human relations. Not that they have been very successful so far! It will take time and the thinking related to it will have to mature.

(e) The individual's future

This concerns the predictable evolution of the individual's motor, perceptive and sensory characteristics as time progresses.

QUESTIONS TO ASK HEALTHCARE AND SOCIAL STAFF

- What residual abilities is the individual likely to have?
- How are they certain, likely or possibly to evolve with time?

  WHY?

- To get to know the extent to which the certain, likely or possible evolutions will impact on objects and environments;
- To understand what can be used, what can be reused with alterations and what has to be replaced;
- To make decisions on the basis of predictable developments (for example, choosing a shower rather than a bath tub or vice versa);
- To draw up a project with a set of milestones:
- Making alterations that do not prejudice probable future developments;
- Doing preventive work, which is simple during construction (for example building walls), but of vital importance for enabling future alterations (e.g. making allowance for supplementary attachments so that the bathroom's layout can be altered in future without having to undertake costly plumbing operations, plus providing plenty of sockets and switches in strategic positions etc.).

(f) The individual's dreams

These are what the individual wants or would like to do, regardless of his ability to do so. They also constitute the individual's idea of himself.

QUESTIONS TO ASK THE INDIVIDUAL

- What unfulfilled or uncompleted objectives did you have that you thought you would have been capable of achieving?
- What objectives do you have now? (Are they the same as before? Have they changed? Or are there new ones now?).

  WHY?

  To get to know what look it would be right to give to a place (over and above catering for material needs):

- Reproducing the past as faithfully as possible? In other words, giving the impression that nothing has changed?
- Preserving the same atmosphere as in the past, but inside an updated and modified home?

- Renewing everything, but paying attention to focusing on the things and situations that are important for the individual?

(B) Getting to Know the Others

Discovering the individual's social relations with the people who live under the same roof.

The others are the people who live with the individual on a stable basis.

The architect or designer has to get to know these others and discover how the family group is made up and the dynamics of how they live together. While the primary source for information remains the individual, that information has to be compared with the others, because the data gathered could otherwise be skewed by the expression of wishes and fears rather than of reality.

The methods for gathering this information are interviews aiming at obtaining answers to specific questions, consultation with third parties and contacts with reliable sources, because those with a direct interest often give a false report about their condition or do not recognise it. One way of learning a great deal is direct observation of spontaneous behaviour.

THINKING ABOUT IT

Many disciplines offer us tools for investigating subjective issues. While this is not the place to go into this in detail, the thing I want to point out is that Design for All does not offer original investigatory tools of its own (except its constant reference to holism), but suggests consciously choosing established methods and tools suitable for achieving the requirements of a design for everyone. No new set of tools, then, but a way of using familiar tools and fine-tuning their application. But note that this does not mean just limiting the tools to questionnaires and interviews, because the contextual observation of users and/or ethnic groups, for example, and task analysis are very effective tools for drawing a real distinction between what is real and what an individual says for the purpose of making a good impression with others. It is often far more effective to ask for a glass of water or a coffee and to observe what getting it for you entails than to ask lots of questions.

(a) With whom does the individual live?

This refers to knowledge about the family nucleus living under the same roof, the formal and informal rules of cohabitation, how they relate to the outside world and to any carers and assistants.

QUESTIONS TO ASK THE INDIVIDUAL AND THE OTHERS

How is the cohabiting family made up? (Does the individual live alone in his family, or with others?);

How are vital activities managed? (Nutrition, hygiene, rest, leisure time etc.):

- completely independently?
- with individual assistance (how and when)?
- with public assistance (how and when)?

WHY?

- To get to know how things really stand.

(b) Who does what?

This refers to knowledge about the domestic activities that the individual under-takes or would like to undertake independently.

QUESTIONS TO ASK THE INDIVIDUAL AND THE OTHERS

What activities does the individual undertake in the home for himself or for the others: cooking (always and for everyone, as the need arises, only small things, never), cleaning (for everyone, only his own spaces, never), washing (for everyone, only his own clothes, never).

WHY?

To get to know what choices have to be made.

The kitchen has to be:

- Specialised for the individual;
- Specialised so as to include the individual, but also cater for the others;
- A place where the individual can do small jobs (e.g. heat up a coffee or fry an egg);
- Specialised for the others, because the individual does not or cannot use it.

Doing the washing has to be:

- Designed to suit the individual;
- Designed so as to include the individual, but also to cater for the others;
- Designed for the others, because the individual does not or cannot do it.

Doing the cleaning has to be:

- Designed to suit the individual throughout the house;
- Designed to suit the individual in his part of the house;
- Designed for the others, because the individual does not or cannot do it.

(c) The individual's affections

This refers to knowledge about the individual's affections and how they are likely to evolve: what personal relationships does he have inside the family nucleus that cohabits with him and with the rest of the family outside the home and how do these influence his life, whether positively or negatively?

QUESTIONS TO ASK THE INDIVIDUAL

What relationships do you have inside the home (this is a thorny subject, because it is very intimate):

- with your family (relationships of affection and intimacy as they exist today)?

- in the past (relationships of affection and intimacy as they existed in the past)?
- in future (perspectives or hopes for relationships of affection in the future)?

WHY?

    To establish whether the house should be:

- Based on islands that do not communicate very much (a completely autonomous zone for the individual);
- Designed around places for socialising (common areas + private areas);
- Completely permeable (a house with no restrictions).

(d) The individual's friendships

The aim of the right question in this case is to find out about the individual's friendships and the people with whom he exchanges help outside his family nucleus.

QUESTIONS TO ASK THE INDIVIDUAL

    What relationships (friendships etc.) do you have outside your family nucleus:

- in your community (village, neighbourhood, local square)?
- with relations who do not live with you (your broader family)?
- with your friends (from work, from leisure pursuits, from an association or political party)?
- from the local bar or pub?
- among your immediate neighbours?
- from institutions you belong to (your local church or community centre)?
- with pets (your own and/or those of others)?

WHY?

    To get to know whether the individual's external social life has an influence on the structure of the house:

- Does the individual want to share it with others?
- Are there any infrastructures installed in it (Internet, a workshop for social activities etc.)?
- Does external social life have no influence on the structure of the house?

(e) The dynamics of the home

This refers to the presence or absence in the home of the members of the group who cohabit there with the individual and the dynamics: expected changes and theorised changes.

QUESTIONS TO ASK THE INDIVIDUAL AND OTHERS

    Describe the daily dynamics of the people who live with you:

- their presence and/or absence in the house in the course of the day;
- their presence and/or absence at weekends.

Describe the annual dynamics of the people who live with you:

- their presence and/or absence during various periods (related to holidays, studies, work etc.).

Describe the possible or probable social dynamics of the people who live with you:

- marriage, childbirth etc.;
- other prospects (grown children leaving home etc.).

WHY?
So as to be able to predict the dynamics of the house:

- Rooms whose use changes as the day goes by (e.g. studying then play, family get-together then individual activities etc.);
- Rooms whose use changes as time goes by (e.g. a bedroom for a guest, a party with lots of friends etc.);
- Rooms whose use changes permanently with time.

(C) Getting to Know the Place

Discovering the limitations and possibilities of the built environment.

Places exercise an enormous influence on the possibilities people have to live and to cohabit. Houses are never just built structures: they are also and principally places that produce limitations and opportunities. You only have to consider how the various rooms are oriented with respect to sunshine at various hours of the day, in the different seasons and as a function of the geographical location. Issues like these are very familiar to any architect or builder, as are all the restrictions set by law and building regulations. They have to be approached from a slightly different stand-point when drawing up a design for elderly people.

(a) The current state of the building

This refers to knowledge about the building's current condition (its interiors, how they relate to the outdoors, its furnishings etc.), with a special focus on any critical elements.

QUESTIONS TO ASK TECHNICIANS
Describe your analysis of the existing situation, providing:

- a metric survey using conventional methods;
- a survey of the interiors (identifying the rooms, their actual purposes etc.);
- a survey of how the interiors relate in general to the outdoors (in terms of climate, noise transfer, accessibility, sightlines etc.);
- a survey of elements that express something about the inhabitants' lifestyles (distribution and characteristics of the furnishings, presence of entertainment systems, bookshelves, hobby equipment etc.);
- a survey of the real use made of places and products on the basis of the marks left by their use.

WHY?

So as to get to know the purposes of the various rooms in the house:

- Acoustic issues caused by outdoor noise levels or by the building's plant systems;
- Natural daytime lighting (how the building is oriented and other aspects of natural lighting);
- Quality of the views (what can you see outdoors?).
- So as to get to know the substance of existing structures:
- The size of the bookcase, as an indication of interests;
- The size of the cupboards, as an indication of needs;
- Other specific characteristics.

So as to get to know the building's current condition and the restrictions set on it by the law and building regulations:

- General laws and regulations;
- Local regulations;
- Rules of the condominium;
- Tax incentives, if any.

(b) Making changes

This refers to discovering the potential of the place, its state of technical readiness for change, what the people involved can afford to spend and their psychological readiness for change.

QUESTIONS TO ASK THE INDIVIDUAL AND OTHERS

- To what degree are the people involved prepared to exploit the potential of the places?
- To what degree are they prepared to overcome the problems arising from the places?
- To what degree can they afford change and to what degree are they psychologically ready for it or likely to resist it?

WHY?

So as to get to know the technical potential of the places in question:

- What new extensions to the building are permissible and possible?
- What alterations and modifications of the building's structures are permissible and possible?
- Are any other alterations possible (e.g. new windows, skylights etc.)?

So as to get to know:

- The economic resources immediately available;
- The economic resources available over time;
- The possibility to spread the alteration work over time (in a complete project that makes provision for execution in several self-contained blocks).
- Propensity to change.

(c) The design project

The design project is a highly complex and creative specialised task that takes place at the end of the information gathering process. Although this process is the prerogative of the designer, it should be the moment when shared ideas and aspirations are converted into tangible reality.

QUESTIONS TO ASK TECHNICIANS, THE INDIVIDUAL AND OTHERS
How can the expectations, the readiness and the restrictions on exploiting the potential for change of places and of catering for everybody's needs be translated into practice? By:

- brainstorming with the individual and with groups;
- defining the aims of the design project;
- developing the metaproject, the phase that translates from concepts to decisions (the metaproject already contains all the solutions, but only in embryonic form).

WHY?

- So as to lay the foundations for an executive project agreed by all interested parties and oriented towards Design for All.

8.5   Away from Home, Like at Home

I feel I have been made welcome.

People have plenty of occasions when they do not want to stay at home. Regardless of whether they have more or less serious difficulties of any kind, many of them may prefer to live in a protected environment, where they feel that someone understands them, welcomes them and maybe spoils them a little. In many cases, the social and working context at home means that individuals' lives would in any case be conditioned by outsiders who care for them on a professional basis.

When elderly people live in a more or less specialised institution or go on holiday, to a spa or on a cruise, alone or in company with others, for a few days or for a longer period, they must be able to get about independently, since this is a right for everybody. They are to be identified as individuals, not as patients, so they do not want the kind of attention they would get in hospital. They want to be able to behave away from home just as they would if they were at home.

Every person with disabilities is entitled to be able to get around alone and to be able to travel in a satisfactory way, together with others who are equally satisfied. The others should not have to feel that they are restricted or obliged by his presence.

When I travel, I must be certain of the reception I can expect.

Who can help me? Who can give me a guarantee that I shall find what I expect and that has probably been promised to me in the places where I go?

I have to find people who know the place and ask them about who goes there, why they go there and what they do most when they are there. As a designer, I have to find people who know about human limitations and ask them what I should do to avoid generating frustrating effects for certain categories of people. I have to find people who know about the most frequent pathologies and ask them what the places can/must stimulate.

Every place has its own vocation.

Unlike private houses, these places cannot be designed for specific individuals, but must be conceived for a general cross-section of humanity, which changes all the time, so also has problems that change all the time. So these places have to be suitable for a general cross-section of cases. The information about them has to come from awareness about their vocation, their specific traits and the opportunities they offer.

Someone is bound to remind me that there is a law covering all this. It's true: accessibility is often the result of laws, but very often we will search in vain for respect for human dignity.

THINKING ABOUT IT

People who have real difficulty in getting around ask for information about how accessible a hotel is before they reserve a room. Reassured, they then arrive and often discover that the room itself is accessible, but not the bar, the restaurant or the garden. "But you didn't ask me about that…" is the reaction at the reception. The implied message is that the guest asked for a room, not the right to enjoy a comfortable stay. Luckily, there are now bodies that check these things on our behalf and give us the certainty that we will get a good reception.

Everyone is different.

Structures that are suitable 'for all' cannot be made to measure for a 'patient', but have to cater for the plurality of needs found in different and unknown people and of all those who accompany them for one reason or another.

Every design must pay attention to the needs of:

- those who are weakest (this is the most fragile category in terms of feasibility, perception and sensitivity of their needs);
- couples, because people must also be able to maintain their links (as a couple or individually) with others who have different problems from theirs, without this constituting an obstacle to the smooth running of their lives;
- relations (whose lifestyles should not be impoverished, but if possible enriched);
- the structure's health staff and others, who must be able to work professionally and calmly for the good of the people being hosted;
- technical staff (who must be able to work safely):

8.6   A Welcome for All

Receiving a warm welcome when you are away from home is a very important issue that can vary as a function of the nature of the place and of the probable duration of the stay: "*generic places*" (hotels, holiday villages etc.) are not devoted to anyone in particular, but must be able to host people with problems even when they travel alone, "*specialised places*" are ones that are purpose-built to host people with generic disabilities (the elderly) or specific disabilities (Down syndrome, blind people etc.), while "*adapted houses*" are ordinary public or private housing intended for people with disabilities.

(A) Generic places

Hospitality for All.

These are the structures that form the fabric of hospitality everywhere, in town and country: hotels, spa resorts, residential hotels, colleges, tourist villages, cruise liners, campsites etc. These structures are devised, built and managed to cater for well-defined, tried and tested hospitality systems.

In order to make these structures DfA, they must be equipped and managed in ways that pay particular attention to people with problems. Not only people with motor or perceptive deficits, but also all sorts of other situations of potential difficulty, such as large families, families with very young children, the elderly etc. To be sure of that the structure's characteristics are inclusive, all this must be certifiable and certified, and this is often the case.

WHAT SHOULD BE DONE?

A project based on Asking the Right Question calls for particular attention to be paid to catering for the physical and perceptive needs of those who have the greatest difficulties, but also focuses on the image conveyed by the final result, which must not feel in any way like a ghetto.

Hotels, for example, should have a lot more rooms 'for people with disabilities' than the numbers set by law, but they should be so attractive that they can be let to everyone.

WHY?

The law decrees compliance with criteria of accessibility and describes them in detail.

In the case of hotels, for example, it stipulate how many rooms it must have for people with disabilities. But it only deals with places' physical accessibility and says nothing about emotive, perceptive and sensory issues. That explains why these rooms often have a discriminating atmosphere (like something in a hospital) and cannot be used 'by all', so often remain vacant, awaiting the 'disabled guest'.

A different design approach that thinks of rooms and bathrooms for all, both accessible and attractive, could make them perfectly acceptable to 'the disabled' but also to people who have no problems (or think they have none).

Such hotels could break into the market with a positive image that makes a strong impact for the high degree of attention they pay to 'all', which could be certified, because if good practices are truly good, they are often practically invisible. The market would benefit doubly, because this would solve particular problems, such as when a whole group of wheelchair users wants to stay together and not distributed between several different hotels, following a logic that certainly has nothing to do with common sense or people's rights.

WHAT SHOULD BE DONE?

These structures have to comply with very detailed and highly targeted legal, technical and market standards. The designer is certainly a specialist: for his work to be classifiable as DfA, he must combine his skills with a particular attention for the methods and the criteria of a DfA approach, by:

- addressing the right question to all those who know the most frequent conditions of physical and psychological difficulty that may derive from living away from home, far from the individual's usual and familiar places and belongings;
- addressing the right question to samples of potential users who have had experiences comparable to what will be offered by the structure (the term 'users' includes all stakeholders: end users, those responsible for services and maintenance, the management and so on);
- convincing the client that the design of the structure's management is not a derivative of the design of its physical attributes (something to be developed only after the physical design has been completed), but that the two designs must be synergic and contemporaneous;
- being prepared to stimulate the management design and collaborate with it, exploiting restrictions that are inevitably set on his creativity by transforming them into opportunities of design innovation;
- choosing details and décor that are original and creative, but do not conflict with the probable users' habits and beliefs (including their religious convictions), and leaving leeway for the personal touch.

THINKING ABOUT IT

In the seventies, I often visited the eastern stretch of the Ligurian coastline for work, where I met many interesting people who told me a host of fascinating anecdotes. One in particular concerned the hospital in Rapallo, which had been obliged to close its A&E at weekends because the fine upstanding Milanese bourgeoisie had developed the habit of taking grandad to the A&E on Saturday morning and collecting him on Sunday evening. The A&E was sure to find that grandad had some problem or other and in the meantime his caring relations could go out on their cabin cruiser.

(B) Specialised places

Assistance for All.

These are structures intended specifically for particular situations (ageing, dementia, physical disability etc.) and for particular purposes (tourism, residence, rehabilitation etc.). These may be family homes, rest homes for the elderly, rehabilitation centres, institutions focusing on certain clear and serious pathologies (such as institutions for people who are both blind and deaf) and so on.

The structure's degree of specialisation may vary, in accordance with the management's objectives. An institution for the blind will obviously focus primarily on the blind, while a retirement home may cater for a wide variety of individuals with different kinds of difficulties.

THINKING ABOUT IT

What happens when the Paralympics are organised? I found myself wondering about this, but failed to get any convincing answers.

Were the Olympic Village and the other Olympic structures so well designed and built that no further adaptations were necessary when the athletes with disabilities arrived? In other words, were they DfA? I have my doubts.

Was the design for the Olympics conceived to be adaptable, so that it was easy for the changes to be made, at least to the structures involved, in the handful of weeks between the Olympics and the Paralympics?

Or did the athletes stay in any space that was accessible (for example on the ground floor) without paying any attention to their need to be together?

If anyone knows, I'd be interested to hear.

WHAT SHOULD BE DONE?

The design should make due allowance for all the features necessary to cater for its users, who in certain cases may also be well-defined and definable categories of individuals. In such cases, there will obviously be a prevalence of certain disabilities that have to be tackled by applying all the specific criteria. But it should be remembered that:

- the places must be accessible to all (residents, those who accompany them and visitors);
- residents must be able to bring their life experiences (or at least symbols of them) into the structure;
- special attention must be paid to the quality of the staff's work.

THINKING ABOUT IT

In the Netherlands, there is a good example of what a 'non-clinic' should be like.

The little village of Hogewey is not far from Amsterdam. It has 23 houses, restaurants, cafés, shops, a beauty salon, a theatre and a cinema. 152 people live there, all of them elderly and all suffering from a serious form of dementia or an advanced stage of Alzheimer's. Hogewey is in fact a care home that's organised as a small village, so that the patients can live an almost normal life and feel at home, while at the same time receiving the care they need. There are CCTVs in all the streets, to keep an eye on the patients, while the gardeners, the cashiers and the post office employees are really nurses and doctors. Altogether there are 250 of them, who monitor the patients' health without the patients realising. But maybe such things only happen in a place like the Netherlands, where a doctor can also ply another trade for the purpose of working seriously as a doctor, without causing a scandal with the trade unions.

(C) Adapted houses

Normal homes for 'normal' individuals.

These are homes that are prepared by public housing authorities or welfare bodies and are intended to be assigned to people with various kinds of disability. They provide the right opportunity to illustrate cases of excellence of how to build virtuously and experiment them tangibly and on a widespread scale.

WHAT SHOULD BE DONE?

Adaptable houses must be devised as examples of excellence across a broad spectrum because they are designed before they are assigned to real individuals with specific problems, so must be able to cater for specific particulars. The design must pay attention to adaptability by providing flexible structures. But these house must never take on the appearance of 'special' houses for 'special' individuals.

8.7   Adaptability

The home also has to be different.

It is very unlikely that structures can cater for all the different requirements of guests that it does not know in advance, unless it accepts unsustainable costs. This means that adaptability must be a primary objective, so that it can be the structure that adapts to the individual and not vice versa.

A DfA approach necessarily includes the application of good design features for all, making the structure suitable for most everyday situations that tend to be critical (according to the criteria of ergonomics, accessibility, self-explanatory interfaces etc.).

Provision must also be made for the application of methods and tools that enable the structure to be adapted also to suit particular requirements, without any special work having to be done. This option could be difficult because of the shortage of systems with a high degree of specialisation that are also attractive and very flexible to use. That market supplies products 'for the disabled' that are nearly always rejected by 'able-bodied' people and often also by the 'disabled' for whom they are intended. A designer may find himself having to invent what he needs: we can only hope that the market will notice this promising opportunity.

WHAT SHOULD BE DONE?

Concepts of flexibility and elasticity must be adopted to tackle the changeable situations that may arise:

- *elasticity in infrastructures*

providing multiple alternative products with different characteristics, for the same usage:

- on the spot, such as when a choice of bed pillows is offered;
- in a remote link, with lists of particular or specialised products described clearly 'in a catalogue' or requested in advance online;

- *immediate elasticity*

which may be applied by anyone as the need arises (flip-top furniture, caster-mounted furniture, hook-on accessories etc.). it must also be possible for the user or his assistant to apply them simply and safely;

- *easy elasticity*

adapting the structure to particular requirements semi-permanently, in a way that can be done without any special skills or knowledge (e.g. inserting or removing a particular bathroom chair or making the kitchen suitable for a wheelchair user). It must be possible for untrained people to do this;

- *specialised elasticity*

being able to make important, semi-permanent alterations to cater for particular requirements (e.g. easily changing the way that rooms are set up as a function of the season or of what people need, just as is normally done in any meeting room). This can be done by people with little training, using no tools or everyday ones.

THINKING ABOUT IT

There are many cases when a design is conceived for generic users and then has to be adapted to a specific one. In 1970, the architect Giancarlo De Carlo discussed how this issue applied to public housing. But tourist villages are also designed for generic users and then have to adapt to the specific requirements of their guests. The right solution would be the 'elastic house' that can be adapted easily by the producer with a handful of elements, by offering an articulated catalogue of solutions designed to cater for many diversified needs, or by the client, who can change the combination of the décor (on request or to suit the season), so avoid decisions that are often difficult to make in advance. The end user may then use everyday elasticity, easily moving furnishings and mobile partition walls, while easy elasticity can be used by unqualified staff (cleaning or maintenance staff), who can make easy adaptations to suit the type of end user in question (a couple with small children, a couple with friends or grown children, young people only etc.) or to suit the changing seasons.

8.8 The Permanence Factor

The longer I stay, the more I must have.

For a system that is capable of predicting and providing for all the most disparate requests possible to be sure to cater also for the particular user of the moment is certainly very complex and expensive and is probably not even feasible. Yet being realistic does not mean risking ignoring the issue. It is possible that a design may call for a degree of adaptation from some people in certain situations, which may or may not be acceptable, according to how long they stay. An individual's incomplete autonomy may be tolerable for a stay of only a few days (e.g. "I cannot make myself a coffee on my own, I have to have it made"), while such incomplete autonomy would be unacceptable for a stay lasting for an entire academic year.

WHAT SHOULD BE DONE?

The activities and abilities necessary to make the changes must also be consistent with the length of the individual's stay:

- *short stay*

For a stay lasting a week or less, as in a holiday home, a hotel or the like, adaptability must be immediate, easy and practical for anyone or for untrained staff. Even at the cost of a slightly imperfect result.

- *longer stay*

For a stay lasting several weeks or months, as in a residential hotel, a student hall of residence, a care home etc., adaptability must be very targeted and accurate, also at the price of adaptations that call for some moderately specialised work (at the level of maintenance staff).

Designing things and situations.

The design must be integrated and must not be conducted as a series of consequences, from the town plan to the management plan. That approach tends to end up burdening the management with everything that is left unsolved in the design as built... and it may be catastrophic, because the construction costs are a one-off, while the management costs are eternal. This means there is a need for a complete budget that includes both construction costs and management costs (note that management is not necessarily a complex or highly specialised issue; it is often just a case of designing and/or adapting the staff's rhythms, shifts and skills). This is often not simple, yet it must become a strategic objective.

THINKING ABOUT IT

One example that will be familiar to everybody can serve as a demonstration of the fact that a good design should generate a system and not just lump together the technical and construction part, the economic part and the management.

The motorways built during Italy's boom years were designed, built and managed by different bodies that had no dialogue. Those who designed the structures focused on technical issues, thinking that management issues would then be tackled by others. As a result, beautiful shrub-lined central reservations were designed and built.

But then those shrubs had to be trimmed. The motorway management found it had to organise teams of many workers whose main job was to keep the traffic flowing safely, while only a few could actually work on trimming the plants: an enormous waste and a potentially dangerous job that also had the side effect of reducing the motorway's capacity to carry traffic for long periods. And all because of silo thinking. As far as I know, Versilia, on the Tuscan coast, is the only place where the beautiful oleander hedgerows now remain.

WHAT SHOULD BE DONE?

When structures are designed, the approach should make allowance for possible changes in the course of time, alterations dictated by the evolution of technology, of standards of living and of needs.

The choice of décor and of finishes has an enormous influence on how a place looks and is used.

It would be commendable if people who spend long periods of time in a place were to be allowed to bring pieces of their own past with them.

8.9 It's Better to Be Ready

Man changes, so a house can also change.

It's always better to avoid unpleasant surprises and be ready when a new house is built. That goes for both new builds and major rebuilds that call for a comparable degree of technical and economic input. It's usually the investment of a lifetime.

But life changes as time goes by and a house must also be able to change. The changes we have to consider are of course the certain ones due to the passage of time (ageing), but also the ones induced by social developments, relationships, needs, habits and the make-up of the family nucleus (including births and deaths).

We have to 'think for today, but also for tomorrow'. That does not necessarily mean that what we think about has to be unpleasant, just how time flows. When you build a new house, you certainly have plenty of problems to think about today, so you probably have good reason to resist thinking about tomorrow. Yet the designer must make you understand that we can work today to ensure that any (probable) future alteration does not involve substantial additional outlay: it will certainly be a lot less expensive and above all it will be possible and more profitable to sell the house in future.

Change is real, beautiful and desirable.

One certain fact is that people get older.

As time goes by, changes in needs and lifestyles are also very likely to come about. Getting pregnant, having a baby, having to house an elderly relative or one who has little autonomy, having a temporary or permanent disability… these are all things that can happen and for which many homes are quite unsuitable.

The answer is to design and build houses so that, when they are finished, they do not become an obstacle to change, but actually facilitate it.

It would be a mistake to think that all you have to do to get a good result is comply acritically with the numerous building regulations, because they focus on the physical side of things, not their meaning. A ramp will certainly enable you to pass comfortably from one level to another, but if it screams that is an infrastructure for the disabled, it will be shunned, primarily by the disabled themselves.

Who can help me?

We don't know the future: nobody can tell us. Nobody knows, for example, whether a second child will be the same gender as the first. And that may mean major changes in the structure of the home. But what we do know is the present and that's a good place to start.

Everyone can be a source of information. First of all, everyone who will live in the house, who can talk about their projects and their aspirations; then the specialists, who can talk about the probabilities of things happening in time or of what usually happens.

But above all you have to count on the skills of architects and designers who have been made aware.

Nobody is standard and the house should also not be standard.

We know about the present. We also need to get to know people's dreams and aspirations.

We build on dreams and on models of probable and possible development: on what will happen and will be positive and also on what is unexpected and potentially negative. A design cannot cater for future needs that are still unknown today, but it can be based on elasticity, so that changes can be made as the need arises. Asking the right question enables the designer to progress from the generic 'good design' to the elasticity of a 'predictive design'.

In order to 'be ready', then, a house must be predisposed to make allowance, if and when the need arises, for important work (such as installing a lift) and must incorporate design features that make it friendly and safe from the start, making it transformable, monitoring the points where floors change level, tackling mobility and safety... in short designing an intelligent house.

8.10   Transformability

Man changes... what about the house?

The first issue to discuss is transformability, which means that it has to be possible to alter the house and adapt it to people's changing habits, needs and limitations. It must also be able to adapt to the changes that technology brings with every passing day.

While many technological changes are a question of fashion, others have become part of how we live. Who could manage a modern lifestyle these days without a cell phone and the web?

Every house should be elastic and transformable to cater both for expected challenges and for the ones that are less predictable, for changes coming from new technologies and above all for changes in individuals' lifestyles and capacities, as they develop in younger people and are consolidated in the elderly.

To find out what requirements of flexibility are expected of a new house, you have to 'ask the right question', addressing it to all the members of the family, in the case of a group that's already formed and cohesive, and to individuals if the group is in the process of being formed, as in the case of newlyweds.

If the *group is already formed* (a family or similar), we can talk about 'moving house' complete with objects, behaviour and affections.

When the family group is already formed, we have a group of people with whom we can dialogue and can use many informal methods to conduct our search for information about their propensities. First of all by talking and trying to establish an understanding. But what people tell you is not always what they really want: very often, they are too concerned with looking good in the interviewer's eyes, trying to say what he wants them to. Even without a degree in psychology, a good designer can get a lot of information by observing how people behave and interpreting the language of their current home. It will be very difficult to convince people who are probably young that they will age—or worse—one day soon enough. This is the greatest obstacle to achieving a transformable house. The fact that the property will certainly be worth more and be in greater demand in future may be the issue that makes the difference.

Or if the group is *a new one*, such as a newly-married couple or the creation of a new family, or one of the many other ways in which a group comes to live together.

When a new family nucleus is created, it can be quite difficult to estimate its new lifestyles, because even the people directly concerned do not know. They can only talk about hopes or dreams. When a family group is taking shape, conversations that put you on a wavelength with the people concerned can help you glean information about their living habits and study each individual's models.

This category also includes cases when nobody knows who will eventually live in the house at the moment when it is being designed, because it will be sold or assigned. In such cases, the only way out is to refer to everyday local culture and circumstances.

THINKING ABOUT IT

The people in question are probably young and/or newlyweds who can at last afford the home of their dreams. They are not going to want a house for old people or the disabled, because they are neither old nor disabled. It will be hard to make them envisage a future of potential problems and understand the concept of the elastic house: this will certainly be the greatest hurdle to overcome. But once they choose to go this way, they must beware of the pitfalls: the architect may be tempted to fill the house with handles and grab-bars ready for the elderly. That's the easiest way, but also the worst. The house he designs should not be for the disabled, but must make allowance for being transformed without costing a fortune.

WHAT SHOULD BE DONE?

What do we mean by elasticity when we are talking about a design? In theory everything. But in reality we have to study how and where we can or must do something.

There are some parts of the home that you cannot touch because they concern the structure (load-bearing elements and floor casts), while others can be altered more or less easily (partition walls, building plant) and everything to do with the décor is extremely elastic. The aim is to delegate as many functions as possible to the elastic décor, for example by using mobile walls or cupboards as partitions, while sliding doors and wall elements are also an important option for transformability.

- *Load-bearing elements*

Architects know that the vertical load-bearing elements (pillars and walls) should never be touched once they have been built. If they are made of reinforced concrete or steel, they are usually not very bulky, while brickwork is more bulky. Obviously, the less these load-bearing elements are bulky, the less restrictions there will be on changes. Houses built in the early twentieth century in Italy often have a central brick-built load-bearing spine interrupted by full-height spaces for the doors. As a result, the house is divided in two, but all the other partitions are made of very thin elements that are relatively easy to modify.

- *Floor casts*

It is hard to alter reinforced concrete floor casts, while wooden or steel floors are easier. The real challenge to alterations comes when they are part of the building's static system and when they contain building plant.

THINKING ABOUT IT

In the seventies and eighties, an interior designer was not a good professional if he failed to create 'attractive' changes in floor level: they looked good and were something of a signature. These days we take it for granted that an elastic house should only have steps where they are strictly necessary. That's because the greatest obstacle to making multi-storey buildings useable is the presence of stairs, which become a barrier as soon as you have any difficulty getting around and become a complete block if you use a wheel-chair. In these cases, an elastic design has to take care *today* of the possibility to insert a multi-storey lift *in future* (including the basement if there is one), considering today's techniques and standards that will also apply to lifts in future. So part of the floor cast must be easy to remove because it is not involved in the building's static system and is not criss-crossed by building plant.

- *Partitions*

Fixed-structure space partitions are the elements that conflict most glaringly with the concept of the elastic house. The possibility to modify them depends on the technology used to build the walls, but also on whether they contain building plant and whether altering them would entail having to do work on the floors, always an expensive process whose results are uncertain. Partitions made using furnishings can be modified very easily, although they tend to be rather poor at soundproofing.

THINKING ABOUT IT

The first thing to do to make alterations to partition walls possible and affordable is to install continuous floors throughout the apartment and then install the partition walls on top of them. This avoids the costly process of patching up the floor, which is often the real obstacle to even the smallest change, such as simply moving a door along. One way to avoid the uniformity of look that this brings is to copy how the desert nomads put a homely personal touch to the simple beaten earth floors of their tents by making widespread use of their splendid carpets.

You can give an apartment different degree of elasticity. It can be 'everyday', something done by the end user, who moves mobile partition walls around as though they were sliding doors to rearrange the layout of the rooms. It may be 'easy', done by generally capable people who make simple changes as a function of changing needs: this might entail shifting around furniture or mobile partition walls, e.g. the kind that are mounted on tracks. Special features that have not yet been developed might enable good soundproofing to be achieved, this being the real Achilles' heel of extreme elasticity. Lastly, it may be 'specialised', when the changes call for alterations to be made also to the building plant. This is what normally happens in offices, but not yet in the home.

- *Finishes*

Finishes (the tactile qualities, consistency and colour schemes of floors and walls) influence our senses of touch, smell, sight and hearing and can make a place friendly or unfriendly. Our sense of touch sends important messages, certainly to blind people, but also to everybody else. That's why we go for wood in the bedroom, because of its soundproofing and insulation properties.

THINKING ABOUT IT

Since fabric flooring (carpeting) is easy to lay and replace, it has been used for years to make changes easily. Considerations of hygiene (and blown-up photos of mites!) have now decreed its demise as a cover-all. Vinyl flooring is just as practical, with the added bonus of being intrinsically hygienic.

The tactile properties of a floor (but also of other surfaces) influence how we perceive a space and its outlines. We all use our sense of touch to find our way around, even without realising it (how do you find the light switch when you go into a dark room?). Blind people are just more aware of it.

Floors must not be slippery, especially any floors exposed to the weather. Any kind of non-slip floor is fine for everyone and at all times (you don't have to use crutches to learn this).

- *Furnishings*

Furnishings are the part of the home that comes into closest contact with man and his body. Many languages refer to furnishings with a word that means 'mobile' or 'moveable', describing their nature as objects that are easy to move and transport. In some cases, both their position and their function can be modified, while others are even more versatile, because they are modular and their units can be combined. If they are also truly 'mobile' (on casters, foldaway, stackable…), the spaces they occupy can also be modified to suit the needs of the moment. The market offers a broad range of this kind of product.

THINKING ABOUT IT

If we use furnishings as partitions (bookshelves, cupboards…), spaces can be altered quite easily, without having to knock anything down.

- *Building plant systems*

A building's plant systems are the most difficult part of the home to modify, especially the plumbing. In order to make the best use of the slope available, the WC cannot be very far from the main drainage. Toilets with a shredding function can only be a resource in an elastic house if a range is designed one day that manages to break free from the obsession with looking like something for emergency situations.

Wi-Fi control systems can also make electric power systems extremely elastic.

THINKING ABOUT IT

The plumbing is always the least flexible part of any house and every change is bound to be difficult and costly. Simple solutions may include making advance provision for the removal of a sanitary fitting (usually the bidet) to increase accessibility in the bathroom. Toilet bowl and bidet combos have not yet found general acceptance, although they could be a solution in such cases. Having all the plumbed fittings on one wall could also help increase the turning space in the bathroom, by moving the opposite wall (the one with no plumbing) slightly away.

To have elastic power systems, the first simple step to take is to build in an abundance of empty tubes during construction, since these will one day enable even important changes to be made.

One major advantage today comes from the distinction between the actual power supply, which requires a physical connection (at least until someone comes up with the possibility to convey power wireless, if that ever happens), and the control system, which can be via a wire or wireless. It is already feasible today to connect all the power sockets up to the mains and entrust their control to Wi-Fi signals.

Domotics is already with us in advanced homes, although it is still an option for the wealthy. But not for much longer! We shall soon be able to control the status of all our appliances remotely, individually or by functional groups. Anybody will be able to switch anything on or off and use applications to control them remotely when away from home. Our children will be reassured that their elderly parents are fine without having to move away from their own homes!

8.11   Differences in Height

Should not be an obstacle for anyone

Homes are often built on more than one floor and individual housing units often have small differences in level that have to be overcome: the front doorstep, a step in the garden and so on. These should not become an obstacle for anyone. Fixed or mechanical structures have to be installed to overcome these differences in level.

THINKING ABOUT IT

Very few shops have level step-free access. In some cases, they are made accessible by adding a little ramp outside on the pavement, complete with a little parapet that complies with the building standards, but only if there is space enough on the pavement. Does that mean that shopkeepers are all evil?

Of course not! It's the structure of the buildings that leaves no space for ramps, even little ones, inside the perimeter of the building. The floor cast on the ground level, like on all the other floors, is surrounded by a load-bearing beam that contributes to the building's static solidity and cannot be touched!

So why do we not insist that these beams are installed lower down, below the level of the outdoor pavement, in new builds? That way we could have accessible entrances in future to shops, houses and maybe even the gate into the private garden of a couple who have aged in the meantime, as we all do in the end.

- *Houses on multiple levels.*

In homes built on multiple storeys, there are substantial differences in level for accessing the various floors, the basement, mezzanines or attics. Such houses of course have stairs (often spiral staircases) and only occasionally have some form of lift. Stairs are generally considered to be sufficient and often are. But one day they may no longer be, and then it will be necessary to make alterations to install some form of lift. And that is never easy if no provision has been made in advance.

> THINKING ABOUT IT
>
> I only have one leg, but I live in an apartment on two floors linked by a spiral staircase. It may sound absurd, but I have several reasons for preferring a spiral staircase to a normal one. First of all, I have a series of handholds within easy reach, since all the handrail supports are very useful for pulling myself up with my arms. Secondly, the space is very tight, so nothing serious happens even if I trip, because I am always close to a wall to rest against. The problem comes when I have to carry anything up or down. If it's a suitcase, I toss it downstairs, or I pull it up step by step with some difficulty. I'll never be able to carry a cup of coffee up the stairs. Nobody has yet come up with a goods hoist for a spiral staircase!

- *Minor differences in level*

The first thing is never to install steps and changes in level just because they look good: it's pure sadism!

Differences in level are often minor, maybe only one step. This should always be avoided, because steps are always an insurmountable obstacle for wheelchair users, but they also create problems for everyone who uses a trolley, a pushchair or a trolley bag or is trying to move furniture. Steps can be hazardous for small children, for anyone who has difficulty getting around, at night, for blind people or those with poor eyesight and for the elderly. A single step may be difficult to perceive: that's when it becomes a really dangerous trap for everybody.

You have to ask the right question if you want to find out which differences in level are essential and why, and what alternatives are available to steps and stairs. You have to ask the technicians, so as to solve any technical issues of differences in level compared to outdoors and the ones made necessary by the building plant, especially the plumbing, which it ought to be possible to overcome without using steps or changing level.

You also have to ask the members of the family group and find out about their current and probable future mobility, with conversations, informal chats and other methods, so as to discover their current and future habits and how they compare with their new home. Because it does not go without saying that the entire house had to be accessible. The attic and basement may be off limits to a wheelchair user, without that being experienced as a limitation. But if that wheelchair user has a hobby that calls for him to go into the basement, it could be an unacceptable restriction. In the USA it would be almost certainly for everyone. So there is no single rule for everyone: you have to learn by asking the right questions.

Small differences in level can be overcome with a ramp (but the 8% slope allowed by the standards is too steep!), although the fact is that even lower ramps (6–8%) may be troublesome for everyone, because they break our walking rhythm.

Ramps can incorporate and/or replace steps and so solve problems of accessibility, but they must not fill the house with 'standard' handrails that make it look like a hospital.

- *Stairs*

Stairs are a well-established functional, social and aesthetic feature.

They can become irremediably disabling if they are the only solution for managing a change in level, which a synergic design should tackle with a plurality of solutions.

THINKING ABOUT IT

When there is no lift in a multi-storey house, the differences in level have to be overcome with stairs that are bound to be an obstacle for anyone using a pushchair or a wheelchair, for example. The purpose of stairs is to reach the various floors, but also to take things, suitcases, bags, babies, breakfast trays or a person who feels ill up or down.

An ordinary staircase can be good or bad. The correct ratio between the tread and the rise[6] facilitates a natural step when going up or down. Stairs with a triangular tread and spiral staircases can be dangerous for everyone. We all need a solid handrail that goes right up to the top step, especially those of us who have difficulty walking, are overweight or are carrying a baby or a tray. But you should always make sure that the handrail is attractive and not intrusive!

WHAT SHOULD BE DONE?

The world is not divided in two: wheelchair users and others. In reality, there is a vast range of nuances of people—who are overweight, have suffered a trauma, are insecure, weak, inebriated and also children—who may have serious difficulties using stairs or steep ramps.

In order to avoid becoming an obstacle, a difference in level must be designed to be easily accessible on foot, on wheels, in a wheelchair, with a pushchair and with a rollator. Multiple solutions should also be designed to work together, such as ramps for everyone and steps for those in a hurry.

THINKING ABOUT IT

It is a good idea to consider that it may one day be useful to install a stairlift: when the time comes, it will be easy if we already thought about it in advance, so that the built structure does not get in the way. I hope that stairlifts will one day stop being designed as aids for people with disabilities and start being seen as part of the Design for All agenda. In other words, they should really be for everyone (it's attractive and it also takes my suitcases and my breakfast tray upstairs, not just my old grandad). The idea is not to use them only if we are disabled, but to make life easier for everyone and at all times. One good reason is because the fate of a mechanism that is only used occasionally is that it doesn't work when

---

[6]Ergonomics teaches us that the correct ratio between the rise and the tread is provided by the formula $2R + T = 63$, where R is the rise in cm and T is the tread in cm.

the time comes to use it, or nobody remembers how to make it work. The world is full of unused stairlifts that gather dust.

Adding a lift to a finished building may be useful or even indispensable. It will be easy enough if prior allowance has been made and part of the ceiling cast has been built to be easy to remove because it is not structurally vital and contains no building plant.

8.12 Mobility/Safety

A house should never be a trap.

The ability to move around easily and safely.

Inside the home, we move ourselves, things, people and animals. The home is also one of the least safe of places and is the prime cause of accidents in Italy, followed by the workplace and then by traffic. The categories at greatest risk are the elderly and children.

To have a home that is friendly to us, it has to be easy and safe to move both people and things. But in addition to being safe, the home should also 'look safe', in other words its safety should also be clearly perceptible. It is not enough to have a parapet: if a mother does not notice it and perceive it as a safeguard, she will never really relax.

Safety in the home is not a matter of opinion! The home should be safe for everyone.

That much said, however, there are sometimes good reasons for accentuating the normal precautions taken for mobility and safety, when certain people's particular characteristics call for special attention to be paid. They do not have to be cases of obvious pathologies: we have all seen houses where someone has improvised a soft cover for the sharp edges of a table when toddlers start walking on their own and their eyes are at the same level as the table-top.

When I ask the members of the family nucleus the right question, my purpose is to find out whether there are or may be any particular conditions among the individuals or their forms of behaviour that have an impact on movement and safety.

I also have to ask health workers to give me more information about how people's behaviour can be harmful to themselves or others in the case of obvious pathologies.

THINKING ABOUT IT

Stairs always tend to be dangerous, especially if they are badly or poorly lit. In theatres and cinemas, steps are lit specifically so that people whose eyes have not yet adjusted to the gloom can pick them out.

Slippery floors are another source of accidents that can be avoided by installing non-slip flooring that stays non-slip even when it is wet. Slippery floors are dangerous for everyone and a real trap for anyone who uses crutches or a stick to get around.

Bathroom and storage room doors that open inwards risk becoming an obstacle for helping anyone who faints, because an inanimate body may block the door and make it hard to open, especially if the room behind it is small.

Sharp edges and protrusions can be dangerous for people with limited or no eyesight, for everyone in the dark, for people who have difficulty controlling their movements and for children who have not yet learned to recognise the concept of danger.

WHAT SHOULD BE DONE?

To ensure that a house will be safe, its design must also pay attention to the details of the rooms and the furnishings. In other words, an accessible house is not a house that has passed the test of the specialist who has filled it with ramps great and small, but the result of a synergic design involving all the aspects of accessibility and of safety: the structures, the furnishings and how the result is managed, because objects left lying around, rugs to trip over, dark zones etc. are just as dangerous as steps.

- *The layout*

Today's houses are far more open than in the past, when the old model of the home applied a mistaken idea of privacy, shielding the 'private' parts of the home from the danger of being seen by malevolent eyes. Old homes were full of small, useless rooms, such as the entrance hall, lobbies, corridors and anterooms. These days, the 'at-a-glance' perception of a home's overall layout enables anyone to use it more easily.

THINKING ABOUT IT

Just think how the kitchen has changed. At one time it was the realm of the mistress of the house, assisted by her domestic staff, and it was taboo to everyone else, closed, separate and hidden away from outsiders. These days, at least in our cities, preparing food is far less complex (many basic ingredients can be bought clean and ready to use) and guests often take part in the ritual of preparation and final cleaning. The kitchen has changed radically: it is not segregated any more.

- *Doors*

At one time, homes were full of doors that were bulky and hard to handle. These days there are a lot less of them. They are certainly used for functions that call for privacy, such as the bathroom, and often—though not always—when sleeping, as well as for limiting the spread of cooking smells.

THINKING ABOUT IT

Doors can be an obstacle to wheelchair users' movements. Building standards provide data about the width of doorways, but say nothing about that width being really and fully accessible. This is not always the case, as for example when a handle protrudes so far that a sliding door cannot be opened up completely.

Opening and closing a hinged door obliges the user to step back while operating it. This may be difficult for some and is inconvenient for everyone. There is a growing tendency to install sliding doors that avoid this problem and also the issue of the bulk of the door left standing open.

Doors can be hard to open and close if it is not immediately obvious how to do so. What signs tell me if I have to push or pull to open or close a door? The hinges are a strong indicator that can tell me which way the door opens, but they are often concealed. The position of the handle can also tell me, but the message it sends is often ambiguous. Now look at doors with an anti-panic handle: they are perfect for emergencies, but are very ambiguous for everyday use, which is (luckily) prevalent.

A door handle must be easy to grip and it must be obvious how it functions. It should also be suitable for people who are not very strong or have limited grip ability.

8.13   The Intelligent House

Benefitting from the opportunities offered by new technologies.

Technology provides us with many tools that can make it easier to manage the home, such as intelligent fridges and washing machines or robots for cleaning the floor. Physical effort seems to be on the way out in the home, too, following in the footsteps of industrial production.

Then there's domotics, an articulated system that enables the various functions in the home to be managed automatically or with a remote control: switching on and off, opening and closing, being alerted to what is happening, keeping things safe etc. We have moved from a world of sense-related events (I can see that the light is on, the window handle tells me whether it is closed, I can see that the alarm system is set etc.) and we are set to move more all the time to one of symbolic or abstract information (as the light is on, I know that the appliance is activated; a display reminds me that I have left the windows open etc.).

THINKING ABOUT IT

What has already happened in factories is now happening in the home: how we dialogue with our appliances is becoming the issue.

The factory worker traditionally used manual tools and felt how heavy things were. If he made a mistake, something would happen in his immediate vicinity: he might crush a finger, for example. In an automated factory there is far less human effort: the worker primarily handles controls and reads displays. But a mistake or a distraction can lead to a Chernobyl moment!

I remember when systems were first installed for workers to control production from large panels: the thinking was that they had to be given notional tasks (such as recording their data every 20 min) just to keep them alert. We called it the Homer Simpson effect and anyone who follows that family's adventures knows what I mean!

Abstraction is now also making its way into the home. That's no problem for IT natives, who probably have more difficulty detecting signals from the real world, but what about the rest of us? The elderly? One firm has specialised in lifesaving communication systems for the elderly, but having made them to measure it found that the elderly themselves often shun them, because they do not want to be classified as elderly.

Issues related to cognition crop up primarily because many people have difficulty understanding how to use and interpret data. The technicians who design these systems often fail to use cognitive models that are suitable for everyone: for non-experts as well as experts, for the condition in which the individual finds himself (anxiety, a hurry, unfamiliarity, inability to move very much etc.), for the ability to reach something, for the individual's visual perception or the ambient conditions of lighting (in the daytime, at night, with glare). In a nutshell, they did not create a product for all.

THINKING ABOUT IT

When system designers design controls and interfaces applying the logic of how the system functions, not of what users need, they are preparing the ground for future problems. The designer tends to locate the function inside a logical structure that is familiar to him, so he thinks it may also be familiar to everyone else, while users have to respond to an immediate need. Just think how often it is hard to use the thermostat to switch the heating on because you have come home early, but you want to be certain that you do not mess up the system's permanent programming.

When washing machines changed over from mechanical to electronic, manufacturers felt they had to provide them with 20, 40 and even more different wash cycles. It was all the rage! But it didn't last. Only a few years later, washing machines came out with the slogan" uses just one control" and that says it all. Domotic systems for the home tend to be archaic because they offer all the system's enormous potential, but on the same level… so simple, everyday functions become mysterious.

So how do we distinguish a product that is well designed for all? How do we choose it from all the market has to offer? It may be hard to choose the right product if all you have to go by is the specifications listed by its manufacturer, because they practically never make allowance for human characteristics and limitations. Once a specific system of usability certification becomes commonplace it will be of enormous help.[7]

Anyone who designs a home must pay great attention even to the simple interphone, which is not just a telephone receiver attached to the wall any more these days, but a complex tool that is certainly useful, but can be mysterious if it is badly designed.[8] These days it is easy to choose on the basis of energy consumption, as there are indicators. Why not write comparable standards for the various levels of accessibility?

You have to ask the right question if you want to know what needs will have to be catered for using new technologies and what needs are still not even being expressed because people believe they cannot be solved (although they will be soon enough).

The members of the family may be able to tell you what individuals know about IT today and above all to what extent they accept it. But what about tomorrow? We can only make an educated guess that coming generations will be far more familiar with IT.

---

[7]One major contribution to this process comes from the Design for All Quality Label, which guarantees that the product or place in question caters for the needs of the various kinds of users.

[8]One of the Design for All Quality Labels was awarded to an interphone, BTicino's Polix-Video, because it features a control and information system that caters for the needs of a variety of categories of users: people who know nothing about it (children or the elderly), those who normally use it (informed adults) and those who are to a certain extent experts (who can program the association of multiple functions).

Domotics applied to the home tackles the issue of security from third parties (break-ins, alarm systems) and of the safety of the residents (such as remote controlling that all is well with a baby or an elderly relative). It tackles home management by remotely controlling a variety of functions (opening and closing windows, managing the lighting, managing household appliances etc.) that are very useful for everyone and essential for anyone who is bed-bound. Lastly, domotics can manage energy saving really well by controlling heating and cooling appliances, also by synergising them with the weather and with other automated functions in the home.

WHAT SHOULD BE DONE?

The designer has a challenge: to identify needs, including the ones that are apparently impossible to cater for, compare them with what domotics can give us today and then apply that to push for innovation in this field, which is still partly immature so still has a long way to go.

THINKING ABOUT IT

It seems to be established now that domotics will spread a great deal, especially as costs fall as a result of its greater diffusion and as equipment improves. When and how is not something we can forecast at the moment, however.

When it comes, it will bring radical changes to how things are managed, such as the possibility to monitor things and ask for help in real time (both useful and reassuring for the person being monitored, but often also for the one doing the monitoring).

When domotics partners with the spread of the smartphone, it opens the door to possibilities that were inconceivable until only recently, such as monitoring places visually and controlling appliances remotely. And this is only the beginning.

The issue that now seems to be the greatest obstacle is how to manage the interface between the appliance and its users, remembering that elderly users often tend to have a preconceived refusal of new technologies. But many are adapting. Thanks to the mobile telephone.

Appendix A

The Mechanical Harp

Luigi Bandini Buti
May 2016

It all happened at the beginning of the fifteenth century, when secular music started its rapid spread across Europe.

Hermann Poll, a learned connoisseur of musical instruments, paid a visit to Alvise Vendramin, the leading craftsman producing harps in the city of Venice.

Hermann had invented what he called a "mechanical harp", but now he had to find a craftsman would could produce it. He had made careful preparations for the meeting and was ready to use his drawings to make a convincing case.

After the inevitable pleasantries, some of them sugary sweet and others keenly probing—after all, Venice was the closest to the Orient of all the cities of Europe—Hermann launched into the speech he had prepared so carefully.

H: Sir, it is certainly not my place to teach that of which you are the unquestioned master... the instrument that was already played so skilfully by the gods on Mount Olympus and how it functions: the harp.

V: To be sure... indeed it is acknowledged by many that our instruments know no peer, not even in the great plains of the Elbe and of the Danube, up there beyond the Alps.

H: As I am sure you know, I have written a little piece about this wondrous instrument to whose evolution you have made such a great difference... and I have also pondered much. In my view, the spread of the harp seems to be hampered by the great skill required to play upon it.

V: There may be some truth in what you say, but it is mastery that sets the skilled apart from those who have no skill. There are also some very prestigious schools that teach the skill of playing it well... and many wondrous melodies have been written for it.

© Springer Nature Switzerland AG 2019
L. Bandini Buti, *Ask the Right Question*,
https://doi.org/10.1007/978-3-319-96346-4

H: Indeed… I can only agree with you… but this instrument calls for strong, agile fingers. A maestro of this instrument once confided in me that, with his advancing age—he was already 35 years old—he began to perceive some difficulty in the correct use of the instrument, since his hands slowly ceased to be supple twigs ruffled by the breeze and became stiff, knotted boughs. It is true that 35 is a good old age, yet a player can still hope for several years of active life. This made me think how useful would be a mechanical harp, easier to use and more commonplace.

V: So you devised a mechanical harp for the aged and the invalids.

H: No, no, not necessarily… but for everyone, even the young, who must not (or do not wish) to have callouses on their fingertips. A harp for everyone.

V: So what would this mechanical harp be like?

Hermann, who had prepared himself well for this question, now drew out some sketches that would help him explain his meaning. Changing his tone, he adopted a more persuasive demeanour, which he trusted would stand him in good stead with the famous maestro of the art of making musical instruments.

H: The instrument is based primarily on an ordinary harp, so would keep the marvellous sounds made by that instrument of the gods. It is in the pizzicato that my design is innovative. Every string, every note, has a hook that plucks it. If there are 46 strings, there will be 46 automatic fingertips.

V: Very complicated!

H: Less than might appear…

V: But then who shall move all those fingertips?

H: Here lies my true invention, of which, if you will allow, I am very proud. Using simple levers, each note is accompanied by a key that can be pressed simply by merely resting a finger upon it. There is no need for long exercises to learn to play the harp, nor to have particularly sensitive fingertips.

V: From your description, it would appear to be a very complicated product to build that will cost much more than a harp.

H: It will certainly cost something more, but not very much.

The discussion was now reaching the crucial point: Hermann would contribute the idea, but the ducats were to come from Vendramin… and ducats have always had more substance than ideas, which are like leaves in the wind.

V: So, what do you expect from me?

H: I would be greatly honoured if you were to take care of the construction of my mechanical harp, to which I have already given a name: the "harpsichord".

V: So I should put my master joiners to work to construct your "harp of chords"?

H: "Harpsichord".

V: "Harp of chords" or "harpsichord": aught does it change. An instrument to allow old people to play the harp too! But how many old people are there who have no harp (although they must have learned to play it somewhere) and want to buy a new one... made especially for old people.

H: But it is not for old people: it will be useful for everyone...

V: So you say! Can you tell me, perchance, how many will buy such a new instrument? How many old people will be interested?

H: I am sure that my design will usher in a musical revolution: it will enlarge the market and make it possible to produce new sounds that have never been heard before.

V: Numbers: I want numbers!

H: Since this instrument is new, I can make no comparisons, nor can I offer all the certainty that a traditional product would give, but it will certainly be an important new development in music.

V: And I should risk my ducats in an adventure that nobody knows whither it will take us? Dear boy, I applaud your enthusiasm, but allow me to be sincere: your "harp of chords" will never know fortune.

H: "Harpsichord".

V: Yes, as you like. But nobody shall want to use a machine to make music. True musicians shall turn over in their graves and, in the best of cases, should you ever succeed to produce this contraption, it will be considered a surrogate for old people and not for those of us who truly love our music. You will see that nobody will ever speak of your fine idea.

H: Yet I believe that it shall be otherwise!

V: Well met! It is fitting that a youth should think thus... I shall talk of this with my lute makers, but do not expect any result.

In Venice, closed within its traditions and the certainty of its success, nothing more was done. And therein lies the moral: if you are already winning, you have no need to innovate. But the same was not true on the other side of the Alps, where someone a little less famous and less of a winner dared to experiment.

And today the best harpsichords (and their degenerate cousin, the piano) are still Made in Germany... and it is no coincidence that one of the producers is called Hermann.

And the same happens to this very day. Instead of ducats, we now use euros, but change is still something that inspires fear in the heart, especially of simple people.

Appendix B

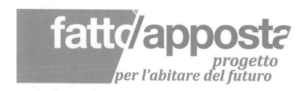

Confartigianato Vicenza 2013–2014

Confartigianato Vicenza, ANAP (the Italian National Association of the Elderly and Pensioners, a branch of Confartigianato) and the Vicenza local health unit N° 6, acting under the patronage of Design for All Italia and involving a series of experts in the field, worked on the issue of active ageing from a perspective of the quality of life and of the habitat.

'Fatto Apposta' (the project's title means 'Made Especially', or 'Custom Made') started out by establishing a multidisciplinary pilot group (businesses working in the home sector, designers and architects, beneficiaries and health service staff) to analyse and share cognitive and design tools for quality habitats for elderly people living alone or in their families, both healthy and recipients of care.

The 'Fatto Apposta' project constitutes a sound foundation for a cultural shift "from care to lifestyle", focusing its attention on the individual and not on his disability.

Participation is the tool that enables a dialogue to develop between the various disciplines and skills necessary for a correct, conscientious design process. Participation certainly does not mean just putting a pencil in a doctor's hand or a stethoscope in the architect's, nor does it mean just asking what the man in the street thinks, as is often the case: participation is a structured working method.

© Springer Nature Switzerland AG 2019
L. Bandini Buti, *Ask the Right Question*,
https://doi.org/10.1007/978-3-319-96346-4

Many disciplines deal with participation in the design process and provide operating tools, but no clear participatory design philosophy (who does what, how, when and with which roles): that is the input that comes from 'Ask the Right Question'.

http://www.confartigianatovicenza.it/progetti/fatto-apposta.

Appendix C

Summary Diagrams to Chapter 8 Active Aging

When you have to adapt an existing home to new needs, that may be traumatic, such as going back home after an important operation, or gradual, such as ageing or quite simply the evolution of the family when a new baby is born.

GOING BACK HOME
I stil feel at home there

GETTING TO KNOW HIM/HER	GETTING TO KNOW THE OTHERS	GETTING TO KNOW THE PLACE
Gathering information about the individuals who need changes to be made	*Discovering the individual's social relations with the people who live under the same roof.*	*Discovering the limitations and possibilities of the built environment*
The individual's needs	**With whom do they live?**	**Current state of the building**
Old needs and new needs	*The family nucleus*	*Surveying the structure and furnishings*
The individual's habits	**Who does what?**	**Making changes**
Old habits and new habits	*Domestic activities done or desired*	*What can you, must you, do you want to change?*
New limitations	**Affections**	**The design project**
Limits of hearing, sight, speech, manual dexterity and memory	*What should the home be like? In units or permeable?*	*The synergic project*
Aspirations	**Friendships**	
Old and new aspirations, real and possible	*What do they want to share and with whom?*	
The future	**The dynamics of the home**	
Residual abilities and how they evolve	*Everyday and seasonal domestic dynamics*	
The individual's dreams		
What do they want and what can be done?		

© Springer Nature Switzerland AG 2019
L. Bandini Buti, *Ask the Right Question*,
https://doi.org/10.1007/978-3-319-96346-4

When an elderly person is in a more or less specialised institution or on holiday, taking spa waters or on a cruise, alone or with others, for an extended period or a few days, he must be able to move autonomously, as this is a right for everyone.

AWAY FROM HOME, LIKE AT HOME
I feel I have been made welcome

TRANSFORMABILITY *Man changes… what about the house?*	**DIFFERENCES IN HEIGHT** *Should not be an obstacle for anyone.*	**THE PERMANENCE FACTOR** *A certain degree of adaptation maybe permissible, according to how long the stay lasts.*
If the group is already formed *(family or similar), we can talk about 'moving house' complete with objects, behaviour and affections.*	**Houses on multiple levels.** *- stairs are considered to be sufficient and often are.* *- a mechanical lift may have to be installed at some future stage.*	**Short stay** *- For a few weeks or less, the place must be adaptable by anyone, even at the cost of some slight compromise with the results.*
If the group is a new one *(a new family nucleus e.g. newly-married) it may be difficult to probe lifestyles because even the people concerned do not know.*	**Minor differences in level** *- Steps create problems for using trolleys and pushchairs, moving suitcases, bags and furnishings.* *- Steps are always an insurmountable obstacle for wheelchair users.*	**Longer stay** *- This lasts several weeks or months: the adaptation must be very targeted, even at the cost of work that calls for specialised interventions.*
Structures *- floor casts are hard to change,* *- partitions with fixed structures clash with the concept of the elastic home.* *- finishes influence our sense of touch, smell, sight and hearing and can make places friendly or unfriendly.* *- furnishings are easy to move.* *- building plant is the most difficult part of the home to change.*	**Stairs** *- Stairs are a consolidated functional, social and aesthetic tool.* *- Stairs can be disabling if they are the only solution for changing level in a building.* *- Changes in level should always be tackled in a synergic, integrated project of multiple solutions.*	

Printed in the United States
By Bookmasters